Advance Praise for *Birth of a New Brain*

"With candid, explicit depictions of her compelling journey through postpartum bipolar disorder, Dyane skillfully brings the painful honesty necessary for growth in our field, as well as hope to those suffering. *Birth of a New Brain* is a rare resource that will benefit practitioners, their patients, and the public at large."

Shoshana S. Bennett, Ph.D.,
Author of *Postpartum Depression for Dummies*,
Clinical Psychologist for Perinatal Disorders

"Dyane Harwood's new book *Birth of a New Brain* is a phenomenal gift to the mental illness community, especially for postpartum sufferers. Dyane's clever weave of gut-wrenching honesty entwined with intricate storytelling illuminates an under-profiled mental illness. *Birth of a New Brain* is an important addition to the world's mood disorder literature, and it will help those with perinatal and bipolar disorders of all kinds. Delve into Dyane's incredible story, one that untangles the baffling and under-reported illness of postpartum bipolar disorder. Prepare to be moved. You won't regret it."

Wendy K. Williamson
Author of *I'm Not Crazy Just Bipolar* and *Two Bipolar Chicks Guide to Survival: Tips for Living with Bipolar Disorder*

"*Birth of a New Brain* is a beautiful portrayal of Dyane Harwood's excruciating journey with bipolar disorder. Her honesty in sharing her grueling experience is impressive and commendable. Our field needs this book. It is edifying and inspiring. *Birth of a New Brain* is a must-read for psychiatric providers and individuals suffering from mood disorders. Dyane's account of her illness is a brave step toward our society embracing the concept that individuals with psychiatric illness deserve to receive casseroles, cards, and flowers, similar to patients with any other medical illness."

Dr. Nancy Byatt, D.O., M.S., M.B.A., F.A.P.M., Medical Director of MCPAP for Moms, Associate Professor of Psychiatry and Obstetrics & Gynecology at the University of Massachusetts Memorial Medical Center and Medical School

"*Birth of a New Brain* by Dyane Harwood is a trailblazing story of hope and recovery. Dyane's depiction of postpartum bipolar disorder will encourage readers who have any form of bipolar disorder to persevere to find effective treatment."

Susan Berger, Chairwoman of the International Bipolar Foundation

"Bipolar illness is serious and widely misunderstood. When it emerges in the postpartum period, women and medical professionals are often blindsided due to the current lack of awareness. Dyane Harwood's *Birth of a New Brain* is a brave and deeply personal account of how bipolar illness can impact a new mother. Dyane's honest reveal of startling references such as mania, ECT, hospital wards, suicide and 'tsunami obsessions' creates heartfelt transparency and highlights its stigma-busting potential. Postpartum women in distress will relate to Dyane's genuineness and be grateful for this book."

−Karen Kleiman, MSW, LCSW, Author of The Art of Holding: An Essential

Intervention for Postpartum Depression and Anxiety, Founder of The Postpartum Stress Center

"This is a story of when love alone can and cannot heal in bipolar disorder. It is a story of mental illness seen through the eyes of a daughter, a wife, and a mother. Dyane Harwood's memoir *Birth of a New Brain* was a privilege to read."

Dr. Greg de Moore, Author of *Finding Sanity: John Cade, Lithium, and the Taming of Bipolar Disorder*, Associate Professor of Psychiatry at Westmead Hospital, Australia

"With artful prose and brutal honesty, Dyane Harwood depicts her struggle to have a stable, peaceful life as a wife and mother amidst the turmoil brought on by postpartum bipolar disorder in *Birth of a New Brain*. Despite many false starts, missteps, and even cruel and indifferent treatment at the hands of certain medical professionals she encountered, Harwood soldiered on and finally arrived at her own truth. The answers, for the most part, were inside her all along and consisted of self-care habits including healthy eating, sufficient sleep, and consistent exercise. Thoroughly researched with a wealth of resources for mothers and families, *Birth of a New Brain* is an invaluable reference point for mothers grappling with shifts in mood after the birth of their children."

Matt Samet, Author of *Death Grip: A Climber's Escape from Benzo Madness*

"*Birth of a New Brain* is a candid portrayal of Dyane Harwood's lived experience of postpartum bipolar disorder. In my 25 years of practice as a perinatal psychiatrist, I have not come across a book that left me so informed and inspired. The mental health field owes her a debt of gratitude for all she has done to highlight the triggering role of childbirth in bipolar disorder. This is fundamental reading for mental health practitioners as well as sufferers of bipolar disorder."

Dr. Verinder Sharma, Professor of
Psychiatry and Obstetrics & Gynecology at
Western University, Ontario, Canada

"With *Birth of a New Brain,* Dyane Harwood adds to the body of work on perinatal mood disorders by providing a thorough, moving account of her journey toward mental wellness after postpartum bipolar mania. Like many other women, because Harwood had no prior diagnosis of bipolar disorder and nobody caught the red flags in her mental history, she was unaware she risked a mental health crisis postpartum. We often associate bipolar disorder (pre-existing or postpartum onset/diagnosis) with postpartum psychosis. Most women with postpartum psychosis may have an underlying bipolar disorder; not all of those with bipolar have psychosis, and not all of those with psychosis have bipolar."

Teresa Twomey, JD, Author of *Understanding
Postpartum Psychosis: A Temporary Madness*

"*Birth of a New Brain* is essential reading not only for mental health care professionals but for anyone who is suffering or knows someone who has been affected by bipolar disorder or a perinatal mood disorder. I admire Dyane for not only sharing her courageous journey but also educating us about a subject that is not nearly discussed enough."

–Lindsay Gerszt, Executive Producer of
When the Bough Breaks: A Documentary

About Postpartum Depression and
Postpartum Psychosis

"Dyane Harwood's writing eloquently brings to life the complex interaction between the person, her world and the changes in how she how she perceives it wrought by the onset of mania following childbirth. She unpicks the conflict faced by all of us who experience chronic mood problems—between the pressure to follow sometimes uncertain 'medical advice' uncritically and the need to retain some sense of self-agency, because with that comes the hope of being able to lead the kind of lives we want to live. She rightly challenges the doctors who project their own failings onto the 'problem patient.' Indeed, she highlights the importance for all of us of finding a doctor in whose expertise one can invest respect and trust. We are all so much more than our 'illness' but can find that goal hard to achieve. Dyane Harwood's extraordinary book shows us how to do it."

Dr. Linda Gask, Author of *The Other Side of Silence: A Psychiatrist's Memoir of Depression*, Emerita Professor of Primary Care Psychiatry at the University of Manchester

"Dyane's journey through mental illness has taken an astonishing amount of twists and turns, and in *Birth of a New Brain*, she generously and courageously shares her experience so that others may learn from it. *Birth of a New Brain* is an invaluable and hopeful guide for anyone confronting mental illness so they can get the help they need and deserve, from professionals and family, without shame."

Mark Lukach, Author of *My Lovely Wife in the Psych Ward*

There is a distinct need for Dyane Harwood's book *Birth of a New Brain*. Although Dyane had a specific trigger for her bipolar disorder, peripartum onset after the birth of her second daughter, her story applies to anyone who has been affected by depression, mania and anxiety, either firsthand or through caring about someone who lives with a mood disorder. Dyane's perseverance in finding treatments and strategies to regain stability will offer hope to those on the same journey, whether they're at the very beginning or somewhere along the way.

Joanne M. Doan, Publisher of *bp Magazine*

"In *Birth of a New Brain*, Dyane Harwood gives voice to countless women who've suffered postpartum bipolar disorder. As a therapist specializing in bipolar disorder, I've seen how this condition can be misdiagnosed and mistreated, especially in the prenatal and postpartum phases. Dyane's passionate story of missed opportunities to correctly identify and treat her mood swings shows us how new mothers can fall through the cracks of a sometimes chaotic mental health system. But her relentless pursuit of the truth behind her anguish gives us hope. Through all the confusion, doubt and despair, she never gives up. Postpartum bipolar disorder is real! And Dyane is an inspiring example of how to thrive far beyond it."

Michael G. Pipich, M.S., LMFT, Therapist,
Author, National Speaker on Bipolar
Disorder

"*Birth of a New Brain* is an important contribution to our understanding of postpartum bipolar disorder. New moms are often unaware that this condition manifests in the complicated ways. Dyane Harwood brings to life with her vivid, compelling prose, and even seasoned clinicians can miss the signs of post-partum hypomania or mania. Dyane brings wit and wisdom to what I think will be very helpful to her peers who experience postpartum bipolar disorder, their loved ones and new families, and the doctors who treat them. In fact, what Dyane so generously shares within *Birth of a New Brain* may well prevent some of the pain and danger that she unfortunately had to experience."

> Allen Doederlein, President of the
> Depression and Bipolar Support Alliance
> (DBSA)

"Dyane Harwood gives voice to the enormous pain and suffering associated with severe postpartum mental illness. In sharing her story of postpartum mania, she poignantly describes the association between bipolar disorder and the exacerbation of symptoms triggered by childbirth. *Birth of a New Brain* is an important book that should be required reading by all who provide care to perinatal women."

> Dr. Samantha Meltzer-Brody, MPH,
> Perinatal Psychiatry Program Director at
> the University of North Carolina Center for
> Women's Mood Disorders

"Dyane Harwood has changed the landscape in our ability to reach out to families and prevent crises related to perinatal bipolar disorders. In *Birth of a New Brain*, Dyane movingly illustrates that the experience of living through the extreme symptoms of bipolar disorders without help is lonely and frightening. Dyane has accomplished a wonderful goal; she not only provides solid information about bipolar mood disorder symptoms, risks, and distress, but also uses her authentic voice to illustrate hope, healing, and stability. Women and families who read this book will come away feeling like they just made a trustworthy friend, one they can rely on for honesty, wisdom, up-to-date facts, and a model of recovery. The book will make a world of difference in the provider's ability to understand risk factors, assess, and support women living with perinatal bipolar mood disorder symptoms, and it will also empower parents to ask the right questions and improve their ability to take healthy steps on the road to recovery."

Wendy N. Davis, PhD, Executive Director
of Postpartum Support International

"In *Birth of a New Brain*, author and advocate Dyane Harwood provides the reader with an intimate look at her journey with postpartum bipolar disorder. This book will be a blessing for anyone who has received a diagnosis of bipolar disorder and wishes they had a best friend to "show them the ropes." Dyane bares her soul and spares no details whether it's describing the effects of myriad medications she was prescribed or the moment she found herself pleading for electroconvulsive therapy (ECT) due to suicidal thoughts. Ultimately, this is a book about hope, courage, and perseverance. I have long admired Dyane as a fellow advocate; after reading this book, I have enormous respect for her as a warrior in the fight against stigma."

–Caroline Whiddon, Co-Founder &
Executive Director of Me2/Orchestra, Inc.

Birth

of a

New Brain

Healing from Postpartum

Bipolar Disorder

DYANE HARWOOD

Foreword By Dr. Carol Henshaw

A POST HILL PRESS BOOK
ISBN: 978-1-61868-801-9
ISBN (eBook): 978-1-61868-800-2

Post Hill Press
New York • Nashville
posthillpress.com

Published in the United States of America

This book is dedicated with all my love to
Craig, Marilla, and Avonlea

"Human neuroscience has shown that a mother's brain changes dramatically during her first pregnancy. The brain's neurons are wired and rewired at a comparable rate to that which occurs during puberty. One can say that a new mother has a different brain than before delivering her child."

> — Dr. Shimi Kang, Author of *The Dolphin Parent: A Parent's Guide to Raising Healthy, Happy and Motivated Kids—Without Turning into a Tiger*

TABLE OF CONTENTS

FOREWORD

Memoirs have been written by women who have suffered from postpartum depression and postpartum psychosis. This book is unusual in that it chronicles Dyane's bipolar disorder from its postpartum onset to the present day. In my clinical experience, it has been difficult for healthcare professionals to recognize hypomania or mania in a woman who has recently given birth. In Dyane's case, no one at the maternity hospital recognized her emerging mania before she was discharged home. Many perinatal psychiatrists rarely address the possibility that postpartum hypomania or mania may signify a first episode of bipolar disorder.

In addition to her postpartum bipolar onset and the heartbreaking separation from her baby during her first psychiatric admission, Dyane looks back at her formative years in Los Angeles, California. Raised by loving parents, her father suffered from bipolar disorder, yet she never imagined she would eventually fall prey to mental illness.

Despite treatment resistance, multiple hospitalizations, electroconvulsive therapy (ECT), a considerable time to find the right medication, and the realization she could not live without it, Dyane has now achieved stability and written a book. This is a tremendous achievement. It is my hope that *Birth of a New Brain* will aid healthcare professionals to improve the treatment of women with postpartum mania after delivery and bipolar disorder subsequently, but above all, I am sure that it will be an inspiration and a source of hope for women in the same or similar situations.

Dr. Carol Henshaw, MB ChB MD
Co-author, *The Modern Management of Perinatal Psychiatry*
Cheshire, United Kingdom

PREFACE

Dyane Harwood's memoir *Birth of a New Brain* may be the single most important book on mental health ever written.

This is an astounding work of heart. Dyane's honesty is staggering. Her story is heartbreaking. Her triumph is overwhelming.

This is the book the mental health community has been waiting for.

Bipolar disorder is so complicated and varied, it's with actual excitement the reader watches Dyane Harwood untangle the ropes of her conditions before they become her noose.

As the reader gets a glimpse of her experiences inside a psychiatric ward and the disintegration of her reality and self, it's difficult not to feel guilty enjoying this book.

Fortunately, Harwood describes the carousel of diagnosis, the cruel gala of mania, and the power of loving vigilance like a best friend describes a fun weekend.

She's not only an author, she's a magician. I will never fully comprehend how Dyane survived, let alone reported back to us, what she saw, felt, and experienced.

From the bottom of my heart, I urge everyone on earth to immediately get this book and share it.

I truly cannot think of adjectives powerful enough to convey the import of *Birth of a New Brain*.

Jay Mohr, Mental Health Advocate,
"Keep Oregon Well" Campaign,
Comedian, and Author

INTRODUCTION

If anyone had told me the birth of my daughter would activate my bipolar disorder, I would have exclaimed, "You're joking, right?"

For most of my life, I thought bipolar disorder, or manic depression as it was formerly called, was only associated with brilliant artists, writers, and actors such as Vincent van Gogh, Virginia Woolf, Robin Williams, Carrie Fisher, and Catherine Zeta-Jones. I certainly didn't think childbirth could activate the mood disorder, especially for someone like me, an average mom who didn't have impressive credentials.

I grew up with bipolar disorder at arm's length. My father, a gifted violinist in the Los Angeles Philharmonic, was diagnosed with bipolar one disorder when he was a young man. Some of his colleagues had bipolar disorder, and he mourned the loss of several friends who died by bipolar-related suicide.

Before my bipolar diagnosis, I worked as a freelance writer. Ever since I was a little girl, I wrote in journals and cultivated pen pal friendships. Writing comforted me. Shortly after I was diagnosed with postpartum bipolar one disorder (now classified as bipolar disorder, peripartum onset by the *Diagnostic and Statistical Manual of Mental Disorders (DSM-5)* used by psychiatrists), I knew I'd be compelled to write about this mood disorder.

Within twenty-four hours of my daughter Marilla's birth, my bipolar disorder manifested as postpartum hypomania, a deceptive symptom because I seemed simply elated, but not to the extreme. In addition to my mania, I wrote nonstop from the moment I returned home from the maternity unit. This compulsion was the rare symptom of postpartum *hypergraphia,* the overwhelming urge to write. Hypergraphia has been linked to the manic state of bipolar disorder and temporal lobe epilepsy.

I never knew hypergraphia existed until I experienced it firsthand. When I was hypergraphic, I wrote so much that my wrist cramped up in agonizing pain. I shook it vigorously to stop the aching, but the pain returned within seconds. I couldn't stop writing for a moment, even when I breastfed my precious newborn or while answering the call of nature! I was caught in a whirl of racing, obsessive thoughts, which is how many people describe their bouts of mania. Instead of noticing my baby girl's sweet scent or feeling her rose-petal soft skin, all I could think was, *I must write this idea down, and this, and this...*

Six weeks after Marilla was born, I was acutely manic. At my husband Craig's urging, I admitted myself to my local hospital's Behavioral Health Unit, a euphemism for the scary-sounding "psychiatric ward." At the unit, I was stunned when I was diagnosed with postpartum bipolar one disorder. Following my diagnosis, I suffered from medication-resistant bipolar depression for seven years, stumbling through my new reality of chronic mental illness.

This is a story about my life before bipolar disorder morphed me into a shadow of my former self. It's an account of the years when bipolar depression made me hopeless, and about how I finally emerged out of depression's tunnel into a healthy, productive (and imperfect!) life.

Many people with bipolar disorder want to relinquish medication. I share my failed attempts to taper off lithium, the gold standard medication for bipolar disorder. Some people with bipolar disorder can live balanced lives without taking medication, but I learned the hard way that I couldn't live medication-free.

After a great deal of trial and error, I've reached a point where my mood is stable. I'm vigilant about safeguarding my mental health. I keep up with research findings as a member of the International Society for Bipolar Disorders and through the internet websites listed in Appendix D: Resources. The internet has also been a wonderful place to connect with other mothers living with bipolar disorder—they encourage me, and a few of them have become good friends.

During the past ten years, I couldn't find a book about postpartum bipolar disorder, the least known of the six primary perinatal mood and anxiety disorders (PMADs). These PMADs are postpartum depression, postpartum obsessive-compulsive disorder (OCD), postpartum panic disorder, postpartum post-traumatic stress disorder (PTSD), and postpartum psychosis. Although postpartum bipolar disorder remains obscure, it shares some of the same symptoms associated with the other perinatal mood and anxiety disorders.

Anyone who lives with a form of bipolar disorder or a perinatal mood and anxiety disorder can relate to my arduous journey. I've been considered the worst-case scenario because I had multiple hospitalizations, took almost every medication under the sun, and I elected to have electroconvulsive therapy. I didn't think it was possible for someone like me to get my life back on track, but I did it. If you suffer from a mood disorder and you're feeling hopeless, my wish is for this book to help you feel less alone in your pain, and give you some suggestions to improve your mood. If you're struggling, please don't give up hope—you can attain mental health and enjoy your life again!

CHAPTER ONE

The Gateway to Postpartum Bipolar Disorder

On a warm August evening, I was heavily pregnant with my second baby girl. I was irritable from the exertion of carrying an extra fifty pounds. I plodded around our stuffy cabin and whined about the pervasive heat. However, my complaints vanished the instant my water broke. As I felt a gush of warm water splash down my legs, I filled up with excitement and trepidation.

"Craig, *Craaaaaig!*" I screeched. "Come over here! She's on her way!"

I was so beside myself that I didn't think I might have scared our two-year-old daughter Avonlea with my caterwauling. I stood in our kitchen in ratty, soaked pajama pants as Craig ran toward me. He took one look at my puddle and called the hospital to see if a room was available.

"Please let them say yes, please let them say yes!" I murmured. A lifelong worrywart, I wanted a hospital room's security and an accommodating staff that would help us if anything went wrong.

"Sounds good, we'll see you soon," Craig said assuredly.

After we had dropped off sleepy Avonlea at my brother Martin's house nearby, we drove to Sutter Maternity Hospital in Santa Cruz, California. Once I was admitted, I stayed up all night in labor, unable to rest because I was in such pain. At dawn, I looked out the window at a large eucalyptus grove, and for a moment I thought we were at a luxurious hotel instead of a sterile hospital. We had splurged on a private room although we couldn't afford it.

"This is déjà vu!" I muttered after a sharp pain reminded me how awful my contractions had been during my first labor with Avonlea.

Although I didn't have postpartum bipolar disorder after my first baby was born, it could have been activated; for some mysterious reason, it was not. My brain wouldn't be primed for bipolar's emergence until I had my second baby. Perinatal psychiatrist Dr. Alain Gregoire, founder of the Maternal Mental Health Alliance, said the postpartum period "carried the highest risk of developing bipolar disorder in the human lifetime," although the reasons are unknown.

Although no one knows what causes bipolar disorder, it's possible my primary triggers were severe sleep deprivation, my genetic predisposition, and hormones, a trio of culprits I'd refer to as the "Trifecta from Hell."

Dr. Christy, a stunning West African physician, was the doctor on call for my regular obstetrician. I hadn't met Dr. Christy during my pregnancy, but when she sprinted into my room two minutes before Marilla took her first breath, I warmed to her beaming smile.

"I can't believe this isn't hurting!" I told her after we made quick introductions. Thanks to an epidural shot, the last few hours of my labor were pain-free. During Avonlea's labor, I declined the epidural shot. I thought I could endure the pain, but it was a decision I regretted.

When babies are born they often hear their mothers' screams of pain, roars of enormous effort, and cries of gratitude. There is the tragedy of a stillbirth when silence or sobs fill the air. Thankfully when Marilla was born at noon, the first sounds she heard were my peals of laughter due to my relief at the absence of pain. Dr. Christy got a kick out of my giggles, and she and I took turns bursting into laughter so loud we sounded as if we had a stand-up comic in the room. I was a superstitious woman, and I believed our laughter served as a good omen. As I cradled the warm new life in my arms, I never suspected I'd soon face more agony in the coming years than I could ever imagine.

During the first forty-eight hours of Marilla's life, obstetricians and nurses examined me at the hospital, and I visited with a handful of close friends. My elderly parents lived four hundred miles away from us in Los Angeles, and they decided they would meet Marilla at my brother's wedding when she'd be five weeks old.

Within hours after Marilla's birth, I became hypomanic. Hypomania is known as the "lesser mania" in the bipolar spectrum. It is a less intense form of full-blown mania. Later, when I became manic, I had most of mania's symptoms listed in the *Diagnostic and Statistical Manual of Mental Disorders (DSM-5)*. These symptoms include an elevated mood, irritability, pursuing goal-directed activities more than usual, heightened energy, a decreased need for sleep, excessive talkativeness, pressurized speech, racing thoughts, spending sprees, hypersexuality, and grandiosity.

I had an elevated mood, I talked a blue streak, and I was so full of energy I felt capable of running a ten-kilometer race. I felt great about myself, which had previously *not* been the case due to my low self-esteem. I couldn't help but feel exuberant over our baby's pain-free debut, but since I didn't have acute mania yet, I appeared normal to everyone around me.

Postpartum hypomania is a misleading condition. A new mother's happy mood doesn't raise red flags. I wasn't psychotic nor was I depressed. None of my maternity center nurses and obstetricians detected my hypomania. Six-pound, big-brown-eyed, adorable Marilla attracted the majority of everyone's attention. As her exhausted, bedraggled mother, I certainly wasn't getting any double takes. During my two days at Sutter Maternity Hospital, I didn't say a word to anyone about how I was feeling.

My fear of being designated an unfit mother made me keep my disturbing thoughts to myself.

In 2007, there was limited social awareness about perinatal mood and anxiety disorders. It wasn't common knowledge that postpartum depression occurred in one in seven deliveries, or that postpartum mania occurred in approximately one or two births in a thousand. At that time the perinatal mood and anxiety disorders were in great need of public recognition as well as widespread detection by the medical population.

Upon our return home, our family members were unavailable to help us, and Craig was busy running his geologic consulting practice. My mother Phyllis gave us the generous gift of paying for a postpartum doula named Salle Webber. A postpartum doula is trained to provide emotional and practical support to the mother during the postpartum period. They tidy up the house, care for siblings, ensure the mother gets rest, prepare meals, and do much more. Salle planned on assisting us the day after we left the hospital. However, she had an unanticipated allergic reaction that prevented her from joining us until four days after Marilla's birth.

Salle hadn't known me before coming to work for our family, but during her first few shifts, she sensed something was wrong with my mental state. I didn't feel judged by her. On the contrary, I could tell Salle was genuinely concerned. Because she had such a caring personality, I loved having Salle help our family. I felt blessed to have this nurturing, wise mother guide us.

In addition to being a doula, Salle was a writer and hula dancer who lived part of the year in Kauai. Avonlea looked forward to her one-on-one time with her "Hula Doula." Craig welcomed Salle's grounded presence, and whenever Salle came over, I felt less frantic. She provided stability and compassion during a fragile time in our lives. Salle had worked with almost two hundred mothers before joining us. While some of these women suffered from postpartum depression, none of them experienced postpartum bipolar hypomania or mania.

Salle's book *The Gentle Art of Newborn Family Care: A Guide for Postpartum Doulas and Caregivers* was published following Marilla's birth. I gave Salle permission to write about working with our family. She referred to me as "Elaine," and candidly described our situation in the chapter on Postpartum Mood Disorders.

Elaine was a bright and talented writer and mother...the first day after the birth of her second baby girl, she became hypomanic. She found herself flooded with images and thoughts. She couldn't sleep, and felt no need to eat. She stayed up all night writing, feeling productive...

When I arrived to help the family on the fourth day, she enthusiastically described this to me. Her body was beginning to crash from the extreme lack of rest and replenishment. This was the beginning of a challenging experience for me, and certainly for Elaine and her family. I spent many hours there, helping her to regulate her energy, urging her to rest, preparing food, and bringing the baby to her when she needed to be fed. I would specifically ask her to sit down and hold the baby for a while, which she loved, but would forget to do. To help control her inappropriate busyness, we would laughingly say "if you can do it in a horizontal position, do it!

Elaine went through bouts of therapy and psychiatry. She and her husband often fought bitterly, especially on weekends when there was no outside help. The level of guilt was high, as well as shame for allowing the children to witness these events. I spent lots of

13

time befriending the older child, bringing stability into her days. The baby began receiving more and more formula, as the father took over nighttime care, or others fed the baby when Elaine was in an agitated state. I found that my devoted attention to Elaine kept her generally calm, and she trusted and confided in me. However, outbursts frequently occurred in my absence, coloring the mood of the home the next day.

Reading Salle's account saddened me, but I knew her book would educate doulas and help mothers suffering from postpartum bipolar disorder. Her explanation reminded me how I wasn't present for those early days with Marilla, Avonlea, or Craig. Despite my sorrow, I valued Salle's clearheaded perspective because I got an objective take on what happened during a time that remains cloudy in my mind. I'll always be grateful for my mother's thoughtful gift of postpartum care. I'm indebted to Salle for being there for my family in such a chaotic setting. Salle wasn't doing her job just for a paycheck—she put her heart, soul, and "aloha" into being our postpartum doula.

During the hours when Salle observed me writing frantically, she was the only person able to persuade me to break away from the computer so I could be with my baby. As perceptive as Salle was, no one knew what had generated my frenzied writing except for one extraordinary woman, and it wouldn't take me long to track her down.

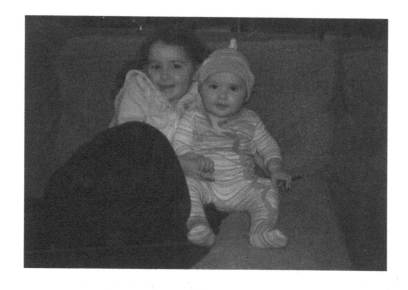

Avonlea and Marilla, Santa Cruz Mountains, California, 2007

CHAPTER TWO

A Crash Course in Hypergraphia

When I was hypomanic, my thoughts raced faster than they ever had before. I related to the character Charly Gordon in the 1968 film *Charly* about a man who becomes a temporary genius. Charly, played by Cliff Robertson, only has superior intelligence for a brief time. When I was hypomanic, I thought of myself as a modern-day Charly because I suddenly felt much more intelligent. I didn't tell a soul about my perception because I realized I'd only sound delusional and pretentious.

Whether or not I had a fleeting genius I.Q., it was evident I had a newfound enthusiasm for life. I was ready to immerse myself in projects I had placed on the back burner such as writing a book and composing songs. I had mixed feelings about my ramped-up brain activity. It was incredible to feel so creative, but my rapid thoughts scared me and made me anxious.

When I returned home with baby Marilla and began writing constantly, I wasn't writing the way I had before her birth. I was prolific to the extreme. I had a compulsive desire to write known as hypergraphia that has been linked to bipolar disorder. My hypergraphic writing behavior was bizarre. I wrote while I tandem breastfed my baby and toddler. I wrote when I was walking around the house and when I went to the bathroom! I wrote on a variety of surfaces such as my hands, the bathroom mirror, inside assorted books, and on my wooden tabletop. I wanted to write down every thought, no matter how insignificant it may have seemed to others. Living with such a heightened sense of urgency filled me with extreme anxiety. My wrists ached from my frenzied typing, and my old carpal tunnel injury flared up. As a result, I was in constant pain.

In theory, hypergraphia seems ideal to writers who suffer from writer's block. The acclaimed author Dr. Alice W. Flaherty reflected upon her hypergraphic experience as positive, but my hypergraphia was bittersweet, with an emphasis on the bitter. Fear was the primary force that drove my writing. Being in a postpartum hypergraphic state was an exhausting way to live.

However, I was in awe that something extraordinary was taking place in my brain. I intuitively knew I couldn't keep up such a frantic pace. All the while, the bullet train of thoughts that sped through my mind prevented me from being able to do much of anything else. I couldn't breastfeed my baby sufficiently, be present with my children, or realize I had the onset of a severe mental illness.

Despite Craig's admonitions that I wrote far too much, I continued to type and handwrite whenever I could. We argued more than we ever had before, and our disagreements took on a nastier tone. Whenever Craig was home, the moment I tapped the laptop keys, our household filled with thick tension.

"Dyane, you need to pay more attention to Marilla and Avonlea!" Craig snapped. I ignored my exasperated husband.

Only a few days had passed since we returned home, and while I wrote, baby Marilla slept and I allowed Avonlea to watch too much television. The postpartum time should have been about bonding with my baby and easing Avonlea into her role as the big sister; instead, I could not give my children the attention they deserved.

My intuition kept whispering something was amiss with my brain. I did a Google search for the phrase "nonstop writing" that yielded various links for "hypergraphia." One link was an interview with Dr. Alice W. Flaherty, author of the book *The Midnight Disease:*

The Drive to Write, Writer's Block, and the Creative Brain. The interview noted Dr. Flaherty's postpartum hypergraphia was depicted in *The Midnight Disease*, and I jotted her name on a notepad so I'd remember to order her book. Next, I reviewed Wikipedia's definition of hypergraphia. I learned it was associated with bipolar disorder, but it didn't dawn on me *I* could have bipolar disorder, despite the fact I had six hallmark symptoms: minimal sleep, racing thoughts, grandiose thinking, hereditary factors, pressurized/ rapid speech, and agitation.

During my sleepless nights, Craig hid my computer so I'd be forced to stop my incessant typing. When my computer vanished, I found an oversized blank book and filled it up with tiny scrawls within two days. After that, I cleaned the house each night. I yearned to have a semblance of order in my life as I organized drawers at 1:00 a.m. I irrationally thought cleaning and sorting socks would help me achieve the equilibrium I desperately desired. I found Craig's hiding place for my laptop in a closet, and I went online to type lengthy emails to friends in the wee hours of the morning.

Night after night I barely slept, yet I revved with energy. I was on the brink of an emotional outburst, but since I did nothing dramatic, no one suspected I was in crisis. It was nearly impossible for me to sit still, and my escalating hypomania affected my ability to breastfeed my baby. At Marilla's one-week check-up, her pediatrician Dr. Austin was concerned with the drop in her weight, and unaware my hypomania was the culprit.

I was running on fumes, and I wanted medical advice on how I could get more sleep. As scattered as I was, I knew I'd get worse if I couldn't break the cycle of only dozing a few hours a night.

While Craig was at a job site inspecting a fault zone, I embarked upon a phone call spree to get help.

First, I called my obstetrician Dr. Moore, and her friendly medical assistant Judi answered the phone.

"Hello, this is Dyane Harwood," I began, my fatigue causing me to slur my words. "I haven't been able to get any sleep! I hate to ask you this, but I need something to help me sleep." As I held my phone with a sweaty hand, I heard other phones ringing in the background, but Judi stayed with me.

"What about an over-the-counter medication?" she suggested.

"I've tried one of those, but it didn't work," I said. "Is it possible to get something stronger?" I held my breath, and waited for Judi to admonish me for wanting a heavy-duty medication.

"I need to get your doctor's approval, but it shouldn't be a problem," she said with no hesitation. I took a deep breath, thankful to get this helpful woman. After we had spoken, she phoned in a prescription to my pharmacy for the medication zolpidem tartrate. For a moment I was proud I had asked for what I needed; assertiveness had never been my strong point, especially when interacting with doctors. I hoped zolpidem tartrate would serve as a magic bullet to break my debilitating insomnia.

Scared and confused about what was happening, I wanted to speak with any mother who had experienced a postpartum crisis. I called a postpartum hotline listed in the phone book, but after dialing the number, a recording announced the line was disconnected. I was incredulous and angry that such an important resource had vanished. I called the maternity hospital's lactation center. (I should have called them in the first place, but my logical thinking was fuzzy.) A receptionist gave me the number of Postpartum Support International's (PSI) California Bay Area hotline.

I reached a PSI volunteer named Linda. She told me she wasn't a licensed therapist, but she would listen and help me however she could. I mentioned my insomnia and fear about calling a doctor for sleep medication. Linda validated my decision to contact Dr. Moore. She advised me to seek local counseling and offered to give me some referrals. We only spoke for a few minutes. I didn't mention my excessive writing or other hypomanic behavior because I was concerned she might report me to Child Protective Services. It was an enormous relief to get advice from a kind, empathetic mother who understood the difficulty of the postpartum time. Before Marilla's birth, I never would have called a hotline or a doctor asking for emergency prescription medication. My hypomania, anxiety, and mothering instinct had sparked my unusual assertiveness.

After I had taken a zolpidem tartrate pill, I got my first decent night's sleep since leaving Sutter Maternity Hospital. The following day, I no longer felt I was about to faint. My sleep pattern stabilized. Craig and I assumed there was nothing to worry about because my hypomania and hypergraphia were subsiding. But little did we know, my bipolar disorder had been activated, and my system was extremely hypersensitive.

At five weeks postpartum, I took part in a celebration that reactivated my hypomania. My brother's fiancé had planned a pampering day with her girlfriends, and she invited me to join them. I wanted to go, but I felt guilty for leaving my girls at home so I could frolic in the wine country. Craig, thinking a change of pace would be good for me, encouraged me to attend, and he offered to take care of Marilla and Avonlea.

Our group planned to meet in San Francisco for a gourmet lunch followed by a limousine tour of several wineries. On my drive up to the city, I stopped at a market to buy a few bottles of champagne for our adventure. I brought my portable breast pump so I wouldn't become engorged, and since I'd be drinking alcohol, I planned to "pump and dump." We drank champagne and wine early in the day and ate plenty of delicious chocolate. During lunch, we drank more wine and gobbled more dessert. It was a feast of excesses, even for me, the self-proclaimed Chocolate Queen.

Throughout the day I had foolishly filled up my body with a massive amount of sugar, not realizing that in doing so, I'd be unable to sleep. Insomnia due to high sugar consumption had never plagued me in the past, but this time around, my tolerance level was radically different. I had become unusually sensitive to sugar. As a result, I stayed up most of the night. My hypomania returned and intensified over the next couple weeks until I was acutely manic.

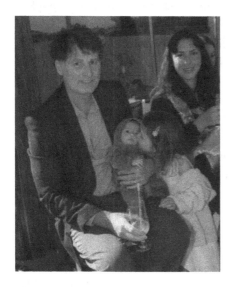

At my brother's wedding five days before my postpartum bipolar diagnosis, October 2007

I was manic when I attended my brother's wedding, but I hid my mania under the guise of being excited. I loved watching my parents meet their easygoing, adorable granddaughter. Marilla was dressed in a brown velvet onesie, and her eyes matched the cocoa color of her outfit. During the celebration, no one took me aside to tell me I was acting manic. I talked constantly, grinned too much, and laughed loudly and often, but it seemed as though I had too much to drink. The focus was on the beautiful bride and handsome groom, not my behavior. Most of the time I sat in the background of the festivities, discreetly breastfeeding my baby.

Unable to sleep a wink the night after the wedding, I had an epiphany at daybreak. I had spent time with my father during the festivities and seeing him brought up memories. One memory was when Dad told me he had stayed up all night unable to sleep because he was manic. At last, I realized I had full-blown mania. I quietly unpacked our laptop and Google searched the internet about "postpartum mania." Once again the name "Dr. Alice W. Flaherty" appeared as it had done when I researched hypergraphia.

Intensely curious, I read a magazine profile about Dr. Flaherty that described her as a brilliant Harvard professor, neurologist, and bestselling author. She lived halfway across the country, but I didn't care where she lived—my goal was to reach her because she understood my bizarre hypergraphic writing *and* postpartum mania, not from a physician or author's point of view but from a firsthand perspective.

Besides being the author of *The Midnight Disease*, Dr. Flaherty was a neurologist at Massachusetts General Hospital. Her book detailed her experience with the tragic death of her newborn twins, her postpartum hypergraphia, and her subsequent hospitalization for what she termed a "postpartum mood disorder" consisting of manic and depressive features. (After her book was published, Dr. Flaherty courageously revealed she had been diagnosed with bipolar disorder in the *New York Times* 2009 profile "From Bipolar Darkness, the Empathy to be a Doctor.")

I found Dr. Flaherty's resume online, and I was surprised it listed her contact information. I couldn't believe my luck! I had the gut feeling this woman could help me. While my family slept in the hotel, I quietly went outside. Dr. Flaherty was in a different time zone, and it was a reasonable hour to call her office. An assistant answered, and as I spoke to her, my speech was rapid and pressurized courtesy of my mania. The assistant asked me to slow down and repeat myself so she could understand me. She promised me she'd deliver my message and called me several hours later to let me know Dr. Flaherty could speak with me the following day. I thanked her profusely.

The next afternoon we were back home. It was an hour before I was scheduled to speak with Dr. Flaherty. I found Craig in the kitchen preparing a snack for the girls.

"I need to talk to you," I said, my stomach in knots. "I'm manic again."

His face crumpled with dismay. "I could tell something was going on, but I'm relieved you're being honest about it. It makes sense to me," he said.

Craig watched the girls when I called Dr. Flaherty's office at 5:00 p.m. She had agreed to give me a brief, pro bono phone consultation. I couldn't believe how fortunate I was. When I spoke, Dr. Flaherty recognized my mania from hearing only two sentences of my manic-fueled speech.

"You need to focus now," she said in a tone of authority. I was embarrassed, but I knew she would give me invaluable advice. From then on, I hung on her every word.

Dr. Flaherty said psychiatric medication had stabilized her postpartum mania. We discussed the aspects of several medications for my symptoms of mania. She didn't suggest I had a specific mood disorder; no ethical physician would ever diagnose over the phone. But Dr. Flaherty strongly encouraged me to see a psychiatrist right away. She urged me to consider using formula as a supplement for Marilla. If I used baby formula, it would enable Craig to do the nighttime feedings and I could get more sleep. We spoke a few more minutes. After I hung up, I was able to sit still and reflect upon the advice I had been given. I was deeply moved this in-demand doctor took time out of her day to help me.

I called Dr. Gordon, a psychiatrist I had consulted when I had clinical depression after leaving a toxic work environment. I wanted him to prescribe olanzapine, a powerful antipsychotic found to subdue mania. Dr. Flaherty had mentioned olanzapine as an option. When Dr. Gordon answered his phone, I lost control of my emotions. Terrified, I sobbed hysterically. I begged him to phone in a prescription for olanzapine so Craig could pick it up the same day.

Through my snorts and tears, I calmed down when I sensed I had Dr. Gordon's undivided attention. I told him about my conversation with Dr. Flaherty and how we had discussed medications for mania, and about olanzapine. Dr. Gordon listened, and he agreed that olanzapine might help quell my mania. After our conversation, he called in an olanzapine prescription to hold me over until we could meet in person.

I took olanzapine the night before Marilla's six-week checkup with Dr. Austin. It didn't work right away. Shortly before we set out for Marilla's appointment, I remembered I wanted to bring the pediatrician a thank-you gift, but I hadn't gotten it yet. In typical manic fashion, I raced around the house looking for anything nice I could re-gift. I decided one gift wasn't enough, so I wanted to find four gifts! I spotted a fancy new vase, a box of Godiva chocolates, and two bottles of wine. Avonlea helped me put the loot in a shopping bag, I grabbed onto the handle of Marilla's baby carrier and we headed out the door.

When Dr. Austin entered the examination room, I greeted him as if I hadn't seen him in years. My booming voice echoed off the walls of the small space.

"Hi Dr. Austin, I have a bunch of *awesome* gifts for you! It's the least I can do to show you how grateful I am! Look at Marilla, isn't she cute? She's the best baby, the sweetest baby, and I'm so in love with her!" I thrust the gift bag at him while Avonlea played with her *Spooky* Halloween book. As he listened to my racing voice and pressurized speech, our UCLA-trained, razor-sharp doctor had a concerned expression.

He looked straight into my eyes and said, "You're manic!"

Although I had done nothing wrong, I felt criticized. I burst into tears. In spite of my humiliation, a sense of relief washed over me. Dr. Austin's assessment meant I didn't have to pretend I was fine any longer. I explained I would be meeting with my psychiatrist, and I had already taken my first dose of olanzapine.

"I'm glad to hear that, Dyane. Everything will be okay," he said as he cradled Marilla in his arms. A few minutes later, Dr. Austin figured out why Marilla's weight had been so low—it was because of my inability to focus long enough to breastfeed her sufficiently. I shook my head back and forth, mortified.

When I took olanzapine, the medication slowed down my racing thoughts, but it wasn't enough—something didn't feel right. My mania wasn't going away. My heart sank when I realized I'd have to leave my newborn, toddler, and husband for medical treatment. I looked at Craig with terrified, watering eyes. My voice cracked as I told him, "I need to go the hospital."

CHAPTER THREE

My Hospital Tour of Duty

When Craig and I agreed that I'd admit myself to the psychiatric unit, I never would've guessed it would be the first of seven hospitalizations.

We used to live in a cabin two blocks from the Santa Cruz Behavioral Health Unit. I had driven by the unimposing, wooden one-story building countless times. The unit was located across the street from the century-old Oakwood Cemetery. I had been afraid of graveyards until we lived next to Oakwood, but I felt comfortable strolling the beautiful, peaceful grounds after work. When I spotted the Behavioral Health Unit on my rambles, I didn't think I'd ever come to know it from the inside.

When Craig and the girls accompanied me to the Behavioral Health Unit, we were asked to wait in the reception room until the charge nurse could begin the admission process. A few minutes later, a thin, curly-haired man walked into the room holding a clipboard. He looked familiar, but it took me a minute to figure out how I knew him. In a strange twist of fate, the charge nurse was Nick, a friend of ours. Craig and I had gone to college with Nick, but we had lost touch over the years, and we had no idea he worked in mental health. It was comforting to recognize a familiar face, and Nick assured Craig he'd keep an eye on me while I was at the unit. When I said goodbye to my family, I hugged Craig tightly. I gave our girls "butterfly" kisses, touching my nose to each sweet face while I blinked my eyelashes against their cheeks. I felt a burst of intense sadness at our impending separation.

Nick asked the receptionist to unlock the doors that would lead us into the women's unit. He promised me he would visit me later, and I was introduced to a short blonde nurse named Sheila. She smiled at me but remained quiet as we walked through the community room. I was surprised there were only a few white-gowned patients milling around.

"Where is everyone?" I asked.

"The patients are in Group Therapy. After that, they'll meet for Self-Care. At noon we break for lunch," Sheila said as we approached a hallway.

Halfway down the corridor, we turned left into a tiny room and faced a windowless space that contained two empty beds. On top of each mustard yellow blanket was a blue folder filled with mental health information and unit procedures. As I set my belongings down, Sheila handed me a toiletries packet, a white gown, and a rough bath towel.

"You'll be meeting with the chief psychiatrist, Dr. King, for your mental health assessment later this morning. You can start group therapy tomorrow. Why don't you get settled, and one of us will get you when the doctor is ready."

"Thanks, Sheila!" I said. After she left, I sat on the bed and stared at the bare, beige walls of the simple room, deflated.

My energy returned when I met with Dr. King. I wasn't embarrassed about my greasy hair, colorless sweatpants and old, grubby t-shirt. Even when I was clean and dressed nicely, doctors intimidated me, but my mania had annihilated my self-consciousness. My appearance no longer mattered. Confidence surged through me—I thought I could take on the world!

We sat down in a sunny alcove in the near-empty community room. The sunshine that poured through two skylights was a contrast to the unit's somber mood. Dr. King could have brought me into a private office, but he made our tête-à-tête casual. I'd come to learn that Dr. King was one of the better psychiatrists who

I'd encounter over the years. He was compassionate, forthright, and knowledgeable. After we had settled ourselves, I turned to face him directly. He spoke in a low, respectful voice. Earlier Dr. King had spoken at length with Craig about my postpartum behavior and my father's bipolar one diagnosis. I was upfront with him about my racing thoughts, insomnia, and hypergraphia, and he heard my pressurized speech.

"Dyane, your symptoms and family history indicate that you have bipolar one disorder. You're in the postpartum stage with your child, and it appears that childbirth was the activating factor. It's a very treatable illness, and if you pursue the proper treatment, then you can live well with it. But finding effective medications takes time, and it can be a matter of trial and error. We can help you start that process here. Do you have any questions?" he asked.

Because I was manic, Dr. King's serious news didn't alarm me. I even found myself smiling. As soon as my five-minute-long, life-changing conversation with Dr. King was over, I made a beeline for the community room's single pay phone. I wanted to tell my father about my diagnosis right away. Since he had bipolar disorder, I knew he'd understand much of what I was experiencing. We had been very close since I was a child when he called me his "Little Dyane," and I wanted to hear his loving voice.

I picked up the receiver and dialed zero to make a collect call. Dad had returned to Los Angeles after my brother's wedding, and in a stroke of luck, he was home to answer the phone. My mania acted as a buffer that prevented me from feeling upset. Now that I was officially diagnosed, my life made sense in an ineffable way. I felt joyful when I picked up the phone to call my father. I was, in fact, experiencing the grandiose thoughts of mania.

Not surprisingly, my father didn't share my elation about my big news. He believed he had genetically passed his bipolar disorder to me, and he felt responsible. I had never seen or heard my father cry until that day. After I told him about my talk with Dr. King, he briefly wept until he was able to speak.

"It's all my fault you have this, my Little Dyane. I'm so sorry," he said. Mania kept me from feeling remorseful about his reaction.

"Dad, everything makes sense now," I said. "Don't worry, I'm doing fine!" I glanced behind me to see a young blonde woman waiting to use the phone.

"Um Dad, someone needs to use the phone. I'll call you later," I said.

"Sure, don't forget! I love you!" he said.

"Of course I'll call back, Dad. I love you too!" I said.

Despite the upbeat sound of my voice and my reassurances, I didn't convince my father I was fine. He knew that my diagnosis was as serious as cancer, diabetes, or any other chronic illness. He didn't want me suffering from the mood disorder.

That initial hospitalization was the only one in which I felt comfortable enough to request visitors. My mania enabled me to be social. I yearned to see familiar faces, especially Marilla, Avonlea, and Craig. My family visited me several times during the four days I was hospitalized.

My mania hadn't made me invulnerable to all tribulations. I was in shock to be separated from my newborn and toddler, and I was homesick. The unit had a jail-like atmosphere that made me feel claustrophobic. Patients weren't allowed outdoors, and there were few windows. I attended Self-Care (during which women applied nail polish from old bottles), Group Therapy (where no one wanted to talk), and Art (where patients colored pictures of simple designs), and I was bored the whole time. During meals, we were given processed food that was beyond recognition and smelled worse than my junior high cafeteria's Mystery Meat.

Suffice it to say, the unit was not on the scale of a high-end facility such as Harvard's prestigious McLean Hospital or Connecticut's Silver Hill Hospital that offered its celebrity clients amenities galore. As each dull day passed, I grew more desperate to leave so I could be a mother again in my home.

My parents offered to visit me, but I didn't want them around while I was in the hospital. I didn't want to hear their bickering and feel their tension when I was in such a sensitive state. There would be opportunities for them to visit after my discharge. My brother was on his honeymoon, and I preferred to let him enjoy it.

There was one person who could give me insider information about the unit. Zachary, my former boyfriend, had been diagnosed with bipolar disorder at the Behavioral Health Unit a few years after we broke up. I called Zachary during his hospitalization and offered to visit him. While he appreciated my gesture, he said the men's section was bedlam. He didn't want me being exposed to the incontinent, fearsome, and violent patients in his unit. I was relieved I didn't go, but I felt bad knowing he was in such a loathsome-sounding place.

When it was my turn to be hospitalized for bipolar disorder, I called Zachary at his company from the pay phone. He was the only person I knew who understood what I was experiencing at the same institution. Zachary was empathetic during our conversation, and he offered to stop by the unit with practical items he thought I'd need. During his visit, he gave me ten dollars' worth of quarters for the pay phone and a bar of lavender soap. More than the quarters or the soap, it helped me to speak with someone who had bipolar disorder and who had experienced the harrowing environment of a psychiatric unit.

Apart from Zachary, my friends Monica, Margo, and Sharon visited me. My co-worker Monica brought a portable breast pump. It was a lifesaver because I had forgotten my portable pump. Inexplicably, the hospital staff never brought me a loaner as they had promised, although the maternity center was across the street from my unit! I was lucky I didn't develop severe mastitis from being painfully engorged with milk.

Margo brought me an exotic treat of fresh pomegranates and gourmet chocolate. As we sat in the community room, the other patients watched us attempt to eat the pomegranates without making a mess. We failed to stay tidy; our faces were covered with ruby red juice, but at least we provided entertainment. I only nibbled on the chocolate since I didn't want my sugar level skyrocketing again.

Sharon was one of my closest friends and had been the maid of honor at my wedding. She brought a Safeway grocery bag filled with women's beauty magazines. Sharon was a gorgeous woman who modeled and sang professionally. When Sharon walked into the community room during our visiting hour, she lit up the place. Heads turned to look at her as she handed me the brown paper bag.

"Dyane, I have some CRAAAAAZY magazines for you!" she sang in her melodious voice.

I couldn't help but laugh at my drama queen friend's Oscar-worthy performance. It was a delightful moment, especially because she drew out chuckles from the other patients. I shared the magazines with them, which they appreciated as they were eager for any diversion.

To help pass the time, I created a lighthearted activity with Morgan, a young female patient who had borderline personality disorder. We developed a television show concept based on our observations in the unit. We christened the series *Boo Hoo*. Morgan and I felt sorry for ourselves that we were stuck in such a gloomy place, and we thought the piteous title was fitting. Discussing wacky *Boo Hoo* storylines kept us laughing in spite of the depressing setting.

After seven hospitalizations, I have scattered bits and pieces of memories from each experience. During my first hospitalization, the hypergraphia had subsided and I was too manic to write anything down in a journal. In my subsequent visits to psychiatric units, I was too depressed to write. My inability to keep a journal spoke volumes about my despondency. Ever since I was little, I used journals to record my sorrow. I found consolation in the act of writing. Lost in hopelessness, I couldn't turn to the one outlet that had given me a respite from my despair.

My hospitalizations had occurred before it was possible for psychiatric units to have internet and cell phone access. I didn't realize it at the time, but being cut off from the internet and from my cell phone impeded my recovery. Although I wouldn't have wanted to speak with anyone but Craig and our girls when I was depressed, I would have listened to friends' messages and read their texts.

When I first became ill, Craig and I didn't have the foresight to search around for an excellent psychiatric program. Although my psychiatric unit environments were grim and the programs were mediocre, I'll never forget that my hospitalizations saved my life. With the growing awareness of the importance of mental health, psychiatric unit programs are improving. If psychiatric hospitalization is required, if possible have a family member or friend research the quality of the program. If the selected unit is farther away from you than other units, it's worth the longer commute to be treated in better conditions. I predict a sea change in the quality of inpatient psychiatric care. While most behavioral health programs won't resemble the opulence of Silver Hill or be affiliated with Harvard, at least there is real hope that psychiatric units will become less sterile and more humane.

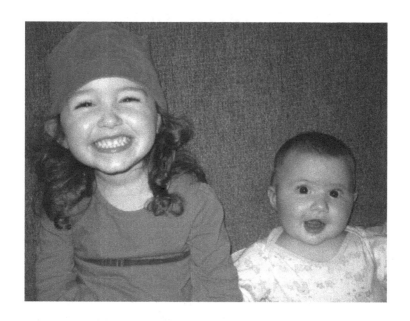

At home with Avonlea and Marilla one month after my first hospitalization,
December 2007

CHAPTER FOUR

California Dreamin'

The desolate environment of the Behavioral Health Unit was a stark contrast to Pacific Palisades, the beautiful California seaside town where I grew up. Pacific Palisades was a place so heavenly that guru Paramahansa Yogananda, author of the classic *Autobiography of a Yogi,* built his Self-Realization Fellowship sanctuary there. The tranquil oasis, located off frenetic Sunset Boulevard, served as a refuge for Los Angeles celebrities who sought enlightenment. Elvis loved visiting the peaceful grounds, and it was the setting for the memorial service of the Beatles' George Harrison. Open to the public, the Fellowship features magnificent Lake Shrine complete with swans, turtles, ducks, koi, lotus flowers, and a windmill. The spiritual feel of the place inspires its famous visitors to forget about the rat race for a few hours.

Many movies and television shows were filmed in Pacific Palisades. The horror movie *Carrie* was shot at Palisades High, my high school—a fact I found quite fitting since I loathed high school! The comedy television series *Curb Your Enthusiasm* was filmed in the Palisadian home of creator/star Larry David. I never set foot on a movie set, but once in a while I'd spot several large Star Waggon trailers parked in front of a house. These trailers served as the movie stars' dressing rooms used on location shoots.

Pacific Palisades has a rich cinematic history. In 1911, film director Thomas Ince revolutionized the motion picture industry. He chose the Palisades Highlands neighborhood for the location of the first major Hollywood studio facility Ever since Ince built his compound nicknamed "Inceville," celebrities made their homes in the area, but my hometown attracted other creative personalities. German and Austrian intellectuals and artists who had been exiled from Nazi Germany in the 1930s and 1940s settled in Pacific Palisades, including Thomas Mann, the Nobel Prize-winning author of *Death in Venice*. When the swinging 1960s arrived, The Beach Boys named Pacific Palisades as a surfing spot in their hit song "Surfin' USA."

In 1970, I was born at St. John's Hospital, Santa Monica, the breezy beachfront city next to Pacific Palisades. I lived with my mother Phyllis, a speech therapist, father Richard, younger brother Martin, and a series of mellow Irish Setters in a home with a spectacular view of the Santa Monica Mountains. My bedroom window overlooked a garden filled with fragrant 'Mr. Lincoln' red roses and robust pink and purple snapdragons. My father was a skilled gardener, and he lovingly tended terraces filled with cherry tomatoes and basil. He was successful in cultivating the land despite its composition of chalky, dense, adobe soil. Dad was well known to the Yamamoto Nursery staff where he bought bags of rich potting soil to mix into his plots.

My father yearned to grow avocado trees, but he could never keep one alive for long. Each time one of his avocado trees died, he was disappointed and frustrated. I didn't understand why he kept trying to grow them, but I found something endearing about his attempts, and I admired his persevering, Don Quixote-esque quest to harvest avocados in his Garden of Eden. I didn't mind our lack of avocados. As a picky eater, I found the green "alligator pear" disgusting, and I wouldn't touch a bowl of guacamole with a ten-foot-long pole. I considered eating a cherry tomato akin to eating a cockroach. I preferred meandering among the rows of flowers, and I loved the scent of our lemon and orange trees when they were in bloom.

Each day I awoke to a view of the Santa Monica Mountain range located several miles north of our neighborhood. I found solace in gazing at the gently sloping mountains. After I got my driver's license, I drove to the base of the mountains, parked near the Los Liones Trailhead, and spent my afternoons roaming the hillsides I had dreamed of exploring.

Now I marvel at my stupidity for hiking alone as a female teenager. I doubt my parents knew what I was doing on my risky excursions, but it was a different time back in the early 1980s when I came of age. Cell phones had not become ubiquitous. My parents often worked long hours during the day and rarely called me. People weren't as afraid of violent crime, perhaps because the internet wasn't around to blast the latest horrifying headlines every minute. The local climate seemed to change overnight when the Los Angeles "Night Stalker" attacks made the cover of the *Los Angeles Times*.

As a girl, I knew I was lucky to live in a place infused with so much natural beauty. I was also fortunate to live in Pacific Palisades before the area was affected by gentrification. During the 1970s, Pacific Palisades was a hidden gem in between Malibu and Santa Monica, attracting movie stars and film industry professionals, but it was still possible for middle-class families to afford to live there. In the 1980s, affluent people from a variety of professions moved into the community, spawning the construction of McMansions devoid of any charm. Obscenely expensive boutiques popped up on every street. Village Books, the only bookstore in town, closed after its loyal customer base dried up due to infirmity or death. No other bookstore took its place, but shops that sold thousand-dollar tank tops and three-hundred-dollar bikini underwear opened for business. While I miss Pacific Palisades, if I had remained there, I would've been disillusioned by how much the town changed for the worse.

As the first child of my family, I was close to my parents during my early years, and I felt adored by them. In the 1970s, I attended

Marquez Elementary School. My parents thought nothing of letting me walk alone for twenty minutes along Sunset Boulevard to reach my school. Although my mother was protective, I was allowed to play with my neighborhood friends with no adult supervision. I never had anything dangerous happen to me, thank God.

My friends and I explored the outdoors often. We hiked the steep, sandy bluffs that edged Asilomar Avenue and overlooked the sparkling blue Pacific Ocean. I rarely invited my friends to play at my house, and preferred to go to their homes instead. I was embarrassed to have visitors due to my parents' fights and my father's depressive spells. When I was ten years old, I befriended a girl named Karen Chanute. Karen had a face spattered with a massive number of freckles topped by stringy, pale brown hair. She was a bookish loner, and lived near me in a rambling California Ranch-style house.

One afternoon Karen and I went to a sand pit located halfway down the bluffs. The kids who knew its secret location were rewarded with access to the powder-soft sand and an amazing ocean view. In our excitement, we jogged to Asilomar, but we started off too fast. Karen stopped for a moment to catch her breath, and I halted beside her.

"My mom said you're a flake," she told me out of the blue.

I thought flakes described snow or cereal, but the critical tone of her voice implied the word meant something else; something that *wasn't* a compliment. Although I didn't know what a flake was, I felt hurt and stopped spending time with Karen. I don't remember what I did to deserve Mrs. Chanute's judgment—maybe I canceled a play date at the last minute, or I didn't show up at her house at all. Although the incident was minor compared to the bullying that I'd experience when I was older, the thirty-five-year-old memory still stings. Rejection during childhood is seldom forgotten.

What Karen and her mother didn't know was that at the age of ten my world was becoming scarier and more confusing. My father was ill with bipolar one disorder and he self-medicated with alcohol. He became ugly and violent when he drank too much red wine. My disconcerted mother was finding out how heartbreaking it was to be married to a man whose mental illness created havoc in our lives. As the years passed, my parents fought more and more. Their quarrels often took place late at night after my father returned home from playing concerts at the Dorothy Chandler Pavilion or the Hollywood Bowl. After Dad walked in the door and set down his violin case, he poured his first glass of red wine and their arguments began.

My bedroom was on the ground floor of our three-story home perched on the edge of Las Pulgas Canyon. My parents' bedroom was upstairs from mine, and I could hear their raised voices through my room's radiator vent. Our home's wooden frame shook whenever they slammed doors in anger. I learned how to race up two flights of stairs in record time so I could prevent my parents from hitting one another. Those evenings were the nightmare underbelly of my life. If Karen's mother knew about my home environment, she might have had compassion for my "flaky" behavior and kept her criticisms to herself.

As I grew older, my mother encouraged me to participate in ballet, gymnastics, and YMCA Palisades-Malibu day camp. Whether I was learning ballet routines at Ebsen Dance Studio or hiking in Temescal Canyon with day campers, I could unwind and forget about the worrisome fights at home. Although the incident with Karen Chanute still rankled, I no longer saw her around the neighborhood or at school. I made new friends with whom I could confide about some of my problems.

When my mother returned to work as a speech pathologist, our family relied upon the indomitable Eva Mae Culpepper, our housekeeper. Eva Mae worked every Friday at our house, and she liked to chat with me after I got home from school. Because of Eva Mae's thick Southern accent, I didn't always understand her, but I tried my best. My mother's training in speech therapy made it easy for her to comprehend Eva Mae's dialect. Mom adored and trusted her, and they became fast friends. They kept in touch after Eva Mae retired in her seventies and remain friends to this day.

Eva Mae had free rein to choose the type of housework she wanted to do, and my mother would never dream of ordering her around. Eva Mae loved to take breaks in our backyard to walk along the terraces and see what was ripe. When Dad was home, she'd ask him if she could take a bag of whatever looked good that day, usually tomatoes. He poked fun at her for "snooping" around, but he was happy she appreciated his produce.

Eva Mae bore witness to my parents' fights, and she often told me, "Girl, your mama and daddy are crazy!" She also had no problem telling me in a matter-of-fact tone that I was "spoiled." Despite my challenge to understand Eva Mae, I heard those observations loud and clear. I knew Eva Mae's assessments of our family were on the nose. My parents were nothing like the even-keeled characters Mike and Carol Brady, the parents I admired on the television show *The Brady Bunch*. I was aware how spoiled I was. I had more advantages than most other kids, but my other friends were spoiled too—we all attended the same extracurricular classes and camps. I felt guilty because I knew every kid deserved such benefits. In any case, I depended upon my after-school programs to take my mind off the violence that occurred at my home.

I was a voracious reader and spent a multitude of hours with my face deep in a book. My mother fostered my love for reading, and in doing so she gave me one of the biggest gifts a parent can give a child. In my mom's family, an appreciation for reading was passed down from generation to generation. Her mother Nettie, my Granny, was an elementary school teacher in 1930s Harlem, New York. Granny was a divorced, single parent, which was rare in that day and age. She was a brave, loving mother of the highest degree, and influenced my mom to become a book enthusiast.

As soon as I could read, my mother gave me thoughtfully chosen books that influenced me significantly such as *A Wrinkle in Time* by Madeleine L'Engle and *Anne of Green Gables* by L.M. Montgomery. I took my books and a flashlight and hid in my bedroom closet, the perfect spot for reading. My hideaway amplified the excitement I found in the world of books.

During the years before I reached my teens, I never understood my father's bipolar illness, nor was I formally told about it until high school. I noticed my father would sometimes hole up in his bedroom on sunshine-drenched days. The heavy curtains that covered my parents' bedroom window were drawn shut, and in the daytime the room was as dark as night. When Dad retreated to his bed in a depression, he reminded me of a bear in hibernation. I felt terrible I couldn't help him out of his misery.

When my father was depressed, he'd tell me I cheered him up. Hearing my Dad say I lifted his mood made me feel special, and I willingly took on a cheerleader role. Yet I remained ignorant about his bipolar disorder. It never occurred to me it wasn't my responsibility to lessen his depression. When I looked at the prescription medications scattered on top of his wooden armoire, I never noticed their names. I never asked him what he needed the pills for, and I had no idea he took all those medications for bipolar disorder and anxiety.

When I attended Marquez Elementary School, Granny retired from teaching sixth grade, and she and her mother Esther moved from New York to Santa Monica so they could be close to our family. Granny loved keeping tabs on how my brother and I did in school, and we spent almost every weekend at her rent-controlled apartment on Ocean Avenue. My sensible, hardworking grandmother was a voice of reason in my chaotic life.

I made a few friends at Marquez Elementary, and some of them had jobs in the entertainment industry. I was friendly with an African-American student named Malcolm-Jamal Warner who, after auditioning for a role on *The Cosby Show*, became famous. Malcolm wasn't a household name when we met, and I got to know him before stardom changed his life. Lindsay Kennedy, another classmate, won a role on the hit television show *Little House on the Prairie*. I had a brush with fame—albeit brief. When I was three years old, my mother brought me to an audition for a commercial. I was told to cry, "There's a fly in my soup!" I must have been convincing because I was selected for the role, but I didn't stop my crying jag after the scene. I took the craft too far, and I was let go from my first job. Thankfully I have no memories of that rejection!

Marquez Elementary had a predominantly Caucasian student body, and when I reached fifth grade, I was placed in a controversial desegregation busing program. I rode a bus to Coliseum Street School in Inglewood, a largely African-American community. While attending Coliseum, I met a student named Kumiko who became one of my best friends. Kumiko was a striking half-Japanese, half-African-American girl who was gifted at playing guitar and writing songs. She lived in an impoverished neighborhood with her devoted single mom, a university librarian, and her loving grandmother. Through my friendship with Kumiko, my eyes opened to the reality of growing up without money. When I visited her small house, I was reminded of Eva Mae's declaration of how spoiled I was, but I would have traded my middle-class perks for Kumiko's peaceful home life in a second.

I was thirteen years old when I was offered my first job. Don was a family friend and a successful optometrist who worked in the Palisades Village. His office manager needed an assistant to label products for sale and do other tasks. I gave the position a try. While I felt proud for doing a "grown-up" job, I found that putting tiny labels on boxes hour after hour was tedious and not worth the extra income. I didn't last there long. Easygoing Don didn't seem to mind when I told him I preferred to be a babysitter.

In junior high during our school's lunch break, my friend Mindy asked me if I was interested in a job. Her mother, a busy modeling agent, had asked Mindy if she knew anyone who was my age and available to work. The job was to pose as the FTD Florist spokesman's daughter in the FTD Father's Day Bouquet ad. The spokesman was Merlin Olsen, the NFL football star-turned-actor.

"You think you'd be up for it?" Mindy asked.

"Sure!" I said, and hoped I wouldn't regret my decision.

I wasn't a beauty destined for a modeling career; in fact, I felt hideous compared to my Barbie doll look-alike classmates. But I was flattered Mindy thought I could pull off being Mr. Olsen's fresh-faced daughter. I wanted to do the photo shoot out of curiosity, plus I wouldn't mind being paid for taking pictures, but what made me seal the deal was that Merlin Olsen was a cast member of *Little House on the Prairie*, and I was a big fan of the show.

When the day of the photo shoot arrived, I was at Granny's apartment in Santa Monica and took a bus to a Culver City studio. The closer the bus got to my stop, the more nervous I felt at the prospect of meeting Merlin Olsen. When I walked into the studio, the set's bright lights made me squint, and I felt intimidated by the strangers who confidently milled about the room. As I was placed into position in front of a flower display, Mr. Olsen walked into the room and stood beside me. I blurted out to him about how anxious I felt. He was gracious and warm, and he set me at ease with humor. I was overjoyed he didn't act like a snobby movie star!

I earned twenty-five dollars for an hour's work, more than twice what I was paid when I babysat.

In a town where most kids my age didn't have to work, I was driven to earn a paycheck. I liked the sense of purpose work gave me, and making money was the icing on the cake. I had saved up a little money towards buying a used car. Like millions of teenagers, I considered driving fun and, most importantly, it allowed me to escape being stuck at home. I felt empowered knowing that if I felt desperate enough, I could escape my parents' arguments. My yearning to have my own car was so strong that when I found out Isuzu was giving away ten Impulse sports cars, I entered the contest five hundred times. I was required to fill out a postcard for each entry, which took a long time. I used my babysitting money to pay for the hundreds of dollars worth of postage I needed. I figured since ten cars were being given away, I had a decent chance at winning the car of my dreams. When I found out I lost the contest, I was bitter for weeks.

After the Impulse fiasco, my mother said she and Granny wanted to buy me a brand-new vehicle because they thought it would be safer than a used car. My generous Granny offered to use her teacher's pension to cover the cost. All I desired was a working set of wheels. Never mind that Mom drove around an old Volvo; it was nothing but the best for her daughter!

Typical Palisadian residents drove flashy Porsches or sleek Jaguars, but my parents drove modest cars. Mom loved the security associated with her banana yellow Volvo station wagon. Dad drove a zippy golden brown Honda Accord LX on his freeway commute to orchestra rehearsals and concerts in downtown Los Angeles. It felt wrong to accept a new automobile when my parents drove high-mileage cars, but the decision had been made. I wasn't going to refuse such a generous gift—I had a strong feeling this would be the only time I'd ever own a brand-new car.

Dad and I drove to the Santa Monica Volkswagen dealership with a blank check. Our young salesperson Mike demonstrated the roominess of the sporty VW Jetta by jumping into a showroom model's trunk and stretching out in it as best as he could. I laughed at his over-the-top selling technique. In a daze, I selected a sparkling dark silver-gray Jetta. When we purchased the car, I sat beside my father at Mike's desk. Dad had notoriously messy handwriting, so he asked me to write out a check for the largest amount I had ever written on any check: eleven thousand dollars. As I held the pen, it was a surreal moment.

I drove my beloved Jetta throughout the Los Angeles suburbs after school and on the weekends. I explored the curvy roads of Pacific Palisades' Castellammare neighborhood that led to my favorite hiking trailhead. I sped along the scenic Pacific Coast Highway to visit Granny for lunches at Polly's Pies on Wilshire Boulevard. Instead of taking the bus, I drove to the Santa Monica Place to meet friends at Vie de France for quiche Lorraine. However, I was forbidden to drive to downtown Los Angeles or Hollywood, areas that were relatively far from my neighborhood. I never broke the rule because I wanted to keep my driving privileges. Moreover, I was scared to visit places known as hotbeds for gangs and other unsavory activities.

When I was sixteen, my father was hospitalized at UCLA's Neuropsychiatric Institute for bipolar disorder. I called him at the unit, and a patient answered the community pay phone. I asked the lost-sounding soul if I could speak with Richard, my father. The patient dropped the phone receiver and it banged against the wall, echoing loudly in my ear. I could hear him yell "Richard" in a haunting, drugged-out voice. It took a while for my father to get on the line, and he sounded groggy and terribly dejected. I thought there must be something I could mention to lift his spirits, and wracked my brain until an answer came.

"Dad, do you want me to bring your violin there?" I asked.

"Sure!" he replied, his voice brightening.

After we had spoken, I located my father's Stradivarius in his practice room. As I picked up the brown muslin case, I handled it gingerly. Antonio Stradivari, the famous string instrument crafter, built the violin in 1685, and I knew it was worth a bevy of Jettas.

The story of how Dad bought his violin is a remarkable one, and it has circulated in music circles throughout the world. During a Los Angeles Philharmonic orchestra tour in Italy, an aggressive peddler approached Dad after a concert. The huckster had gotten backstage and convinced Dad to look at a violin with a beautiful sound. For five thousand dollars the violin could be Dad's. My father declined, but the man wouldn't take no for an answer. He kept after Dad to buy the instrument, and followed him to several more concerts. At last Dad caved and shelled out the money. He was satisfied with his purchase of the modest violin, not to mention relieved he wouldn't have to see the peddler again. Later, Dad had the instrument appraised in London by one of the world's top violin dealers and was told he made the "deal of a lifetime" in purchasing an authentic Stradivarius!

I carefully placed the violin case in the backseat of my car and strapped it down with a seatbelt. I worried about my father as I drove on Sunset Boulevard, and lost in thought, I drove too fast. It only took me twenty minutes to reach UCLA's bleak Neuropsychiatric Institute building. After locating Dad's unit in the directory, I walked up the stairwell and my footsteps echoed forebodingly. My clammy hand clutched the handle of his violin case, and beads of sweat formed on my upper lip.

As soon as I entered the locked-down facility's reception room, my stomach felt queasy. The air felt too cold, and it smelled stale. I believe these places hold energies, and I'm certain the mental health units have absorbed enormous amounts of patients' despair and fear. Although Dad's hospital was affiliated with a top university, his unit appeared second-rate. The walls were dingy white, and there were no pleasant pictures or plants in sight. The medical staff entering the area had grim expressions. The receptionist took one look at Dad's violin case and interrogated me about its contents. She tersely informed me there was no way my father could have his Stradivarius violin in a psychiatric unit.

"What were you thinking? That violin could get damaged in ten seconds!" she sneered.

Chagrined, I realized she had a point. The violin was worth a million dollars. When I embarked upon my Stradivarius mission, I was ignorant that someone in the unit could harm his precious "fiddle," as Dad called it. I didn't realize my father was with patients who were oblivious to their surroundings, or violent— patients who could crush the piece of sixteenth-century wood in a heartbeat.

In the 1980s there wasn't much public education about psychiatric unit protocols. Most sixteen-year-olds were focused on clearing up their acne instead of visiting a parent in a "Cuckoo's Nest." Looking back at that unnerving day, I'm glad I attempted to deliver his violin (despite almost being responsible for its demise). At least Dad knew I tried to help him feel better, and that meant the world to him. Although it didn't work out with the Stradivarius, I was able to sneak in a pack of my father's Trident peppermint gum. He enjoyed chewing it because his medications made his mouth dry.

Back then I had an intense fear of the mentally ill. I never thought I'd have a mental illness, let alone be hospitalized in units similar to the ones my father stayed at during his life. If someone had told my sixteen-year-old self about my future bipolar disorder diagnosis, I would have been more likely to believe I'd become a movie star instead of being diagnosed with a severe mental illness.

My father's diagnosis wasn't discussed in any depth by anyone in our family due to stigma and lack of social awareness. Meanwhile, I was glued to watching "video jockeys" who promoted rock videos on the brand-new music television channel MTV. I loved going to the beach, playing Atari video games, and cruising shops in Westwood with friends. I never heard teachers discuss mental illness at my schools, and I didn't have any friends who mentioned having a parent with a mood disorder, let alone themselves.

During that time, if I had been asked to give a definition of bipolar disorder, I wouldn't have been able to do it. Ironically, I walked through the same high school hallways as another student who would become one of the most respected bipolar disorder authorities in the world. This student was Dr. Kay Redfield Jamison, the author of the bestselling memoir *An Unquiet Mind* and Co-Director of the Mood Disorders Center at Johns Hopkins Medicine.

As the years passed by, I didn't learn much about mental illness. Based on observing my father's blackout days in his room, I had a concrete example of what depression looked like, but I didn't understand his manias in the least. My mother rescued him from the consequences of his reckless, manic actions and depressive collapses. An eloquent, persuasive writer, she wrote letters to his conductors about his mental health, imploring them to save his job in times of his acute depression or mania. If not for my mother, my father would have been fired. Once when Dad was manic, he bid on a $30,000 violin at an auction and won it, but he didn't have the money to close the deal. Mom came to his aid and begged the auction house for mercy, which she received due to her tenacity and charm.

My father's depressions frightened and disturbed me to no end. I felt it was my mission to bring a smile to his face and I worked extra-hard to get him to chuckle when he felt down. Whenever Dad fell into a depression, it wasn't easy being around his pain as I was extremely sensitive. I'd absorb his sadness to some extent, but it was a powerful ego boost for my fragile self-esteem when my father said I brightened his tough days.

I had moments in which I was certain that the darkness that enveloped him would someday smother me. When those worrisome thoughts intruded, I'd ask my father, "Will I get *it*?" I wasn't even able to utter the term "manic depression," and "bipolar disorder" hadn't entered the 1980s vernacular. Each time I asked my father if I'd fall prey to his illness, he replied soothingly, "No, Dyane, there will be a cure for it someday. I promise you won't get it. Don't worry!" I couldn't help but believe his reassuring words.

Inspired by the director John Hughes' teen romance films such as *The Breakfast Club* and *Pretty in Pink*, I pined for a boyfriend. With a teenager's naïveté, I thought my loneliness and fears would dissipate if I found someone who could make me happy. When I was in high school, my math tutor Doreen introduced me to Matthew, a certified public accountant six years older than me. Matthew appeared to have his life together; he had a University of California degree, and he worked full time.

Matthew was lonely too. We spent time together on weekends at his Brentwood apartment, and I began an unhealthy pattern of placing my self-worth and happiness upon being with a boyfriend. This behavior would ultimately backfire when the end of each of my relationships triggered severe depression.

It was unusual for parents to allow their sixteen-year-old daughter to date a grown man, but my mother convinced my father to give his permission. Matthew's mother died of cancer before we met. Mom brought Matthew under her wing, and she was very kind to him. While I was glad they got along so well, I found it off-putting they had deeper conversations than he and I had. While Dad tolerated Matthew, he seldom interacted with him. Dad's precarious mental health kept him from paying much attention to my relationship with my boyfriend. I was no longer my father's little girl, and Dad and I grew distant. It would be years until we returned to our previous level of closeness.

When I was in tenth grade, I spent a lunch hour playing basketball. While dribbling the ball, I pivoted and felt something rip in my right knee. I crumpled to the ground in pain. In a panic, I went to the doctor's office, but I wasn't given tests that would be automatically given today, such as magnetic resonance imaging (MRI) used to create images of tissues within the body. I was told I tore my knee's anterior cruciate ligament. The nurse gave me a list of strengthening exercises for the quadriceps muscles that would help stabilize the knee joint.

I visited the Pacific Palisades YMCA's weight room and learned how to use the free weights and machines. Weight lifting helped alleviate my knee pain and I liked feeling stronger. I ran on the cross-country team before my injury, and I was able to continue running, but I had to stick to shorter distances. Both weight training and running helped me cope better with my turbulent family life and my demoralizing high school experience.

Despite chronic knee pain, I continued exercising to lower my growing anxiety. High achieving students surrounded me in our Advanced Placement classes, their sights set on becoming doctors and lawyers, but I didn't have their drive. I was college-bound, but I was clueless about what I wanted to do in school. I suspected if I had a fresh start away from my father's illness and my parents' acrimonious arguments, maybe I'd figure out my purpose in life after all.

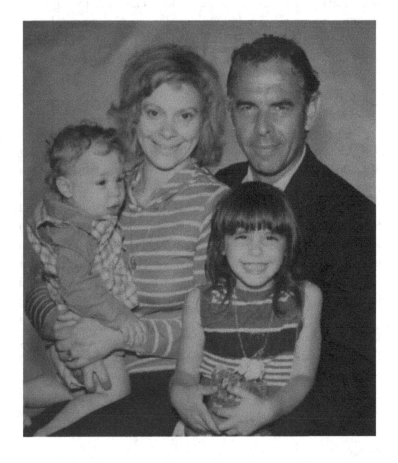

I convinced my nonplussed parents to let me hold my live bug collection for our family portrait. Los Angeles, California, 1977

CHAPTER FIVE

Loneliness and Literature in Santa Cruz

When the time came to apply to colleges, thoughts of my father and his mental illness fell by the wayside. I applied to four schools affiliated with the University of California: Los Angeles, San Diego, Santa Barbara, and Santa Cruz. I hoped I'd get accepted into UCLA so I wouldn't have to move away from Matthew, but my low SAT (Scholastic Aptitude Test) math score destroyed my chances of getting into UCLA.

After much deliberation, I selected U.C. Santa Cruz (UCSC), a college located three hundred miles north of Los Angeles. The distance between UCSC and my family would give me much-needed independence. While my new school's reputation wasn't Ivy League-caliber, I didn't mind. From its 1960s inception, UCSC was known as a hippie mecca. The university was doggedly trying to overcome its negative image through a revamped, rigorous academic program, and I liked the fact that change was in the air. I got a kick out of the university's mascot: a goofy-looking, bright yellow banana slug. I was glad UCSC's administration wasn't afraid to have a sense of humor.

The campus was in a breathtakingly beautiful area of central California and minutes away from the Pacific Ocean. To get a sense of my future home, I visited Elyse, a UCSC freshman who had been an older friend of mine in high school. We explored the vibrant town of Santa Cruz beneath the university but we spent most of our time on campus. UCSC emulated the University of Cambridge and had ten residential colleges. Each college had a unique theme and a distinct appearance, and freshmen were required to live in one of the residential colleges during the first year.

Elyse had chosen Kresge, UCSC's most eclectic college that was known for attracting artsy students and psychology majors. When she took me on a Kresge tour, I was mesmerized by its modern, whimsical architecture and the seemingly random placement of buildings that had been carefully placed to avoid removing redwood trees. The heady environment could pass for a summer camp, and I could see why UCSC had earned the nickname "Uncle Charlie's Summer Camp." Kresge gave me my first taste of how collegiate life was gloriously free of parental restrictions. I wanted to move to UCSC as soon as possible!

During the summer before I left for college, I saw the vampire blockbuster *The Lost Boys* at Westwood's Mann Village Theater. The Mann was one of the world's best movie theaters, and it was used for red-carpet premieres. The theater's enormous screen and the state-of-the-art sound system made any film extra-vivid. Many scenes in *The Lost Boys* were filmed in Santa Cruz, and the film's location scout did a fantastic job at showcasing Santa Cruz's natural beauty. I couldn't help but smile when I realized I was moving to the "Vampire Capital of the World," well, at least according to *The Lost Boys*!

It would be a bittersweet leave-taking because Matthew and I decided on having a long-distance relationship. Nevertheless, I couldn't wait to move into my Santa Cruz dormitory. My enthusiasm helped me sidestep my anxiety about moving far away from my first love.

I spent hours comparing UCSC's ten colleges, and my instinct told me I was making a wise choice when I settled on Cowell College. It was the most traditional college out of the ten, and it had an incredible view of the Monterey Bay. During my freshman year,

I lived in a converted lounge room with three other girls. A bunk bed was tucked into each corner; the top bunk was for sleeping, and the bottom bunk served as a desk. At first, sharing the room didn't bother me, but soon the layout became claustrophobic. My roommates were friendly, but we took different classes and I wasn't close to them. To lower my stress from the demanding curriculum and homesickness, I ran and lifted weights at the school's East Field Recreation Center. Only a two-minute walk from Cowell, the track overlooked the shimmering Monterey Bay, and I always felt a little better after I exercised.

I applied for an off-campus weekend job to distract me from my loneliness, earn money, and give me a break from the stuffy lounge. I was a chocolate fanatic, so I thought a bakery job would be ideal. The student job center listed an entry-level position at Kelly's French Pastries. When I walked into Kelly's, I was met with the enticing aroma of fresh-baked baguettes and French roast coffee. I interviewed with plenty of enthusiasm and landed a counter job. My hourly pay rate was five dollars with no benefits, but I created a job perk. I took full advantage of my access to Kelly's desserts. Employees were forbidden to take home the delectable goods, but I ignored the policy because when chocolate was involved, I threw ethics out the window! I couldn't resist stuffing my backpack with everything the bakery sold except for cakes and coffee.

I convinced my artist friend Jeanette to sell me her hand-painted, green-and-black polka-dotted Honda Spree scooter and helmet with the money I saved from my high school jobs. My eye-catching moped allowed me to reach Kelly's in time for my 5:00 a.m. shift. The Spree maxed out at twenty-five miles per hour. Although it only took twenty minutes to reach the warm bakery, the commute seemed longer because it was icy cold during the early fall and winter mornings. A chilly breeze rushed towards my exposed face, causing me to spill tears as I putt-putted down the hill to Santa Cruz's Pacific Garden Mall.

When I reached the bakery, I walked into the large kitchen where I spotted a steel pot of fragrant chocolate truffle batter; not a soul was in sight. I grabbed a spoon and discreetly helped myself to a bite, making sure not to double-dip because I still had integrity. I made a point of sampling the French pastries during my short breaks so I could inform customers about the exquisite selections. At the close of each shift, I'd fill my backpack with flaky chocolate croissants, blueberry scones and whatever else caught my eye so I could ingratiate my roommates with my spoils.

From the moment my shift began, I sold countless cups of the bakery's French Roast coffee. From my position behind the counter, I peered through the large windows and watched the locals stroll by as they enjoyed the weekend. The most curious standout was known as "Rainbow Ginger," an elderly woman who dressed up in rainbow colors, sported a knee-long scarf, and waved a tambourine. I watched her sing, dance, and kick her leg up high whenever she felt moved to make a spectacle in front of the bakery. (I had no idea this Santa Cruz legend was the great-aunt of my future husband!)

I only worked at Kelly's for a few months and quit because I was tired of waking up so early. Leaving my bakery job was in my best interest because if I remained there, I would have been caught pilfering the yummy goods. Besides, I would've kept devouring too many French treats. I already gained the typical "freshman fifteen" pounds, but I was on my way to gaining a freshman forty. A year later, the ferocious 1989 Loma Prieta earthquake struck at 5:04 p.m., and the bakery and surrounding courtyard were demolished from the damage. Bookshop Santa Cruz was across from Kelly's. The bookstore's brick walls collapsed, crushing a young woman and young man to death at the adjacent Santa Cruz Coffee Roasting Company.

The earthquake registered a 6.9 on the moment magnitude scale, the system used by the United States Geological Survey to measure large earthquakes. I was living off-campus in a second-floor apartment when it occurred. I found the force so terrifying I slept in my car that night. I didn't trust my flimsy 1950s apartment building because I feared it would crush me in an aftershock. Every Los Angeles earthquake I had experienced was a hiccup compared to the violent power of the Loma Prieta. My college education now included firsthand knowledge about how earthquakes caused unimaginable damage and tragic loss of life.

I was sheltered from mental illness during my four years of college. None of my roommates exhibited symptoms of a mood disorder, and my bipolar disorder was latent, not ready to erupt for another twenty years. At UCSC my friends and acquaintances had nothing more serious than mild forms of anxiety or depression. I must have known people throughout college who had mental illnesses, but they didn't dare discuss them because the stigma was far worse in the late 1980s than it is now.

My remarkably generous Granny insisted on using her savings to pay for my college education. I didn't have to work during school and bypassed a pressure that could have triggered my mood disorder. All in all, I was fortunate I had a full college experience untouched by the manifestation of bipolar disorder.

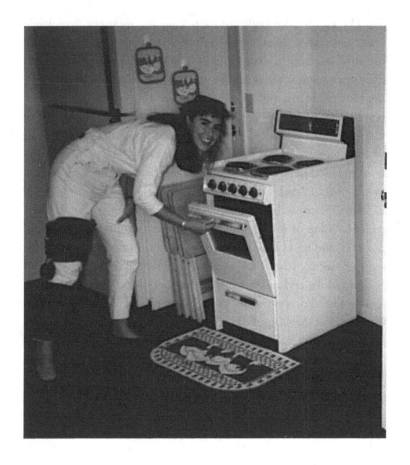

Wearing a knee brace and a phony smile, I'm heartbroken after my knee surgery. Santa Cruz, California, 1991

CHAPTER SIX

Puppy Love and a Broken Heart

During my sophomore year, I invited three classmates to rent a dilapidated house. We moved off-campus into a Palo Alto millionaire's forlorn rental that was in dire need of repairs. The penny-pinching landlord refused to fix anything, but our group was lured by the scenic West Cliff Drive location. I was familiar with West Cliff Drive's cinematic history—it was the location used for the memorable opening credits of *The Lost Boys*. I jogged on West Cliff Drive's walking trail that bordered the ocean. The exercise, invigorating sea breeze, and dazzling view acted as an ideal incentive to get me to work out regularly. As a result, my mood was more level than it had been during my first college year.

Matthew and I continued our long-distance arrangement, and to no one's surprise, we had grown apart. During my second year of college, Matthew called me one evening.

"I've been thinking about it, Dyane. I'd like to move to Santa Cruz. We could rent an apartment, and I know I could find a job," he said.

"Okay," I answered flatly.

Matthew had never left his hometown to attend college, and he was burned out on Los Angeles. His father had passed away the previous year, and he had no other family members in the area. I couldn't blame him for wanting a fresh start in picturesque Santa Cruz, but it troubled me that he overlooked my tepid reaction.

We gave living together a try, but our differences increased. Matthew had found a high-pressure finance job he despised, and his enthusiasm for life was sucked out of him. Sharing an apartment brought out the worst in us, and we broke up after my third year of school. Our split was horrible, but this would be my only romantic demise in which I didn't plummet into a debilitating depression.

Instead, I experienced acute loneliness. I kept busy looking for another place to live, and I discovered how competitive it was to find affordable student housing. After checking the UCSC housing office's bulletin board, I struck gold and found a studio loft in the Santa Cruz Mountains. Once the flurry of moving was complete, my lonesomeness increased. On the rebound from Matthew, I believed a new boyfriend would erase my pain. As I settled into my new surroundings, I became friends with Eric, a young man who lived in a house on the same property as my studio. He shared a home with several housemates, and he had a beautiful Sheltie dog.

When Eric hinted he was interested in me as more than a friend, I was flattered. I gravitated to his offbeat sense of humor and ignored the fluttering red flags that whispered, "This guy isn't right for you." I threw caution to the wind, and we became a couple. I bonded with Chica, his sweet dog, and spent my free time hanging out with her. I had forgotten how much a dog's unconditional love added to my life. I envisioned having a dog and told Eric of my dream to have a furry, four-legged companion.

I procrastinated on taking further steps, but then during the fall, Chica became pregnant. After a smooth gestation period, her labor wound up being awful. Chica crawled into Eric's closet and howled in distress. Frantic with worry, I accompanied Eric and Chica to the veterinarian's office. We learned she would need a cesarean section in light of her precarious physical state. Chica gave birth to a litter of three puppies. When the smallest pup emerged, I looked at Eric. I wanted to care for this tiny survivor and shower her with my love. Eric nodded his head, and my spirits soared. I called her "Tara" after the Buddhist goddess of compassion, a soft-sounding name I had always loved.

I had a blast taking my exuberant puppy on walks, but the additional exercise took a toll on my body. I had searing knee pain that stemmed back to my high school knee injury. I had a sinking feeling my knee pain would only get worse.

In my senior year at UCSC, I moved out of my studio and into Eric's room. I had hoped the greater proximity to my boyfriend meant our relationship was growing more serious, but I was only fooling myself. Although I spent more time with Eric, he kept his emotions to himself, and I wasn't sure how he felt about me. I focused on my increased school workload to distract myself from our problematic relationship.

On a sunny spring afternoon in the Cowell College courtyard, I graduated with a degree in English and American Literature. It was a heat wave and I poured sweat beneath my black cap and gown. When I spotted my family in the audience, joyful tears filled my eyes. As I walked a short distance to receive my diploma, my knee hurt so much I limped. It was a wake-up call, and I realized I couldn't keep putting off a doctor's appointment. It was high time to see an orthopedist, but instead of making an appointment, I drove to Eric's mother's home in Colorado.

Going on a road trip with our dogs in tow was also the perfect excuse to drag my feet about what to do with my life. My mother had helped me financially since my graduation, but she insisted I work to support myself. Upon our return, I planned to substitute teach as a stopgap measure. I felt guilty and ashamed to be a college graduate who didn't have a long-term course of action.

Once Eric and I had arrived in Colorado, I took Tara for a walk and my knee buckled in pain. I could barely make it back to Eric's mother's house. Cell phones were uncommon back in the early 1990s, and I didn't own one. When we returned to Santa

Cruz, I called the office of Dr. Wainer, an orthopedic surgeon. He recommended I have surgery to fix my anterior cruciate ligament and torn cartilage. I wasn't able to walk a step without feeling shooting pain and scheduled the surgery.

Dr. Wainer was friendly and optimistic about my prognosis. The surgery went well, and I had a working knee again! However, everything else in my life fell apart. Hours after I awoke from surgery, Eric visited me in my hospital room. He carried a bouquet of wildflowers and sat down on a chair by the door. Something was off from the moment he arrived. He had an odd half-smile and a detached air that hinted he wasn't there to deliver good news.

"Dyane, I can't be with you anymore," he said casually as if he told me he was going to the market.

As soon as I heard his words, I pressed the self-administered morphine medication button, but morphine wouldn't be enough to soothe my heartache. During the past year, Eric's behavior made me feel he was embarrassed I was his girlfriend. I didn't feel like we were a couple. To make matters worse, Eric would be the first person to leave me to be with someone else. Months before my surgery, I had met Michelle, an exotic blonde-haired dancer, at a social gathering. Eric stared at her as if he were a hungry dog eyeing a meaty bone. I felt a strong twinge of jealousy, but I remained in denial that he and Michele were more than friends. As I lay helpless in the hospital bed, Eric announced he was getting together with Michelle.

As tough as my breakup with Matthew had been, at least it was a mutual split. It was entirely different to be dumped for someone else, especially when I couldn't walk. I felt crushed by Eric's rejection. That day marked the beginning of my first major, undiagnosed depression.

A few hours after Eric's visit, a hospital-affiliated Catholic nun came to see me. After I tearfully told her of my heartbreak, she took one look at me and said, "At least Jesus loves you!" The well-meaning nun's assurances were cold comfort, especially because I wasn't Catholic—I was just a highly sensitive person prone to depression. But I believe having a strong faith would have made me more resilient, and it could have mitigated the depth of my anguish.

This situation was a blessing in disguise because I did myself a great disservice during my time with Eric. Although we had been together for two years, he never told me he loved me. Ever since I was a child, if I loved someone, I always told that person "I love you!" without reservation. Eric's reticence was anathema. His aloof behavior took a toll on my spirit and chipped away at my confidence, yet I was too frightened to leave him. I didn't have enough self-esteem to believe I could find another man who could tell me he loved me, and whose actions supported those words.

What made our split particularly difficult was that I was on crutches for several weeks after my knee surgery. Eric told me I could take as much time as I needed to move, but I wanted to get out of there as soon as I could! My fellow substitute teacher friends Linda and Frances felt sorry for me. When they offered to pack and move all my belongings, I was grateful more than I could express in words. I had located a studio rental on the Westside of Santa Cruz. The landlords asked for a ridiculously high amount of rent, especially given that the "studio" wasn't a studio per se. It was a tiny room containing a countertop, ancient mini-fridge, and a Lilliputian bathroom. On the bright side, I was thankful my landlords allowed Tara to live there, although there was no fenced-in yard. Since it was difficult to find dog-friendly rentals, I signed the rental agreement in the hopes I could find something better for Tara when I could walk without crutches.

My mother continued helping me financially with no deadline, but with the expectation I'd stop accepting her assistance as soon as I could. My father, who was enjoying a time of mood stability, drove to Santa Cruz for a few days to cheer me up. He stayed at a motel down the road and took me to Riva Fish House, an excellent restaurant on the Santa Cruz Wharf. We ordered Riva's mouthwatering snapper ravigote, but I couldn't eat more than a few bites. My Dad grew alarmed when I could not eat a spoonful of the chocolate gelato dessert—I had a reputation for never turning down any opportunity for chocolate!

My father encouraged me to make an appointment with a therapist, unaware I had a deeper problem other than a young woman's broken heart. I perfunctorily agreed I'd find a therapist after his trip. I was touched by his love and effort to visit me, but since I was depressed, I could barely speak when we were together. It was a reversal of our usual roles, and I grimly noted the irony of the situation.

If I could have exercised after the breakup, it would've undoubtedly helped my depression. Instead, I sat around while my knee healed and reached out to others through old-fashioned letter writing. I joined a pen pal club for the rock group Crowded House. I had listened to the Antipodean band's albums for years, but I didn't know anyone who liked their music. The club put me in touch with a young man named Zachary. He felt the same way about Crowded House as I did, and we exchanged letters.

Zachary was also in his early twenties and lived in New Jersey. He worked at an Atlantic City casino and had a large family. Zachary was a funny, engaging, and gifted writer. We found out we both liked to write songs and play guitar, and together we composed a song called *Surprise*. We took turns recording our contributions, and our demo cassette tape flew back and forth from coast to coast. *Surprise* was a romantic song, and after a few months had passed, I realized I felt attracted to Zach despite never having met him in person. It was easy to idealize a stranger and imbue him with the qualities I wished Eric had possessed. When Zachary hinted in a letter at having romantic feelings for me, I thought our pen-pal friendship had the potential for a real-life relationship. We phoned each other and spoke for hours, racking up large bills that drained our bank accounts.

Once my knee healed, I was thrilled to move out of the studio for Tara's sake and mine. The room had reeked of a sickly sweet odor caused by a decaying rodent in the walls. The landlords didn't take care of the problem. Ignorant of my tenant rights, I didn't know I could have called the UCSC Student Housing office for free advice. I wanted to leave the smelly, nauseating room as soon as I could.

Now that I was crutch-free again, I was in a much better position to find an affordable studio that welcomed dogs *and* was stink-free! After combing the newspaper classifieds, I found a rental in a historic building behind a seashell pink Victorian house. The studio had probably been part of a carriage house for storing coaches and other vehicles in the early 1900s. The landlord Patricia and I had an instant connection. I liked her even more when she told me the rent was within my budget! One of the studio's advantages was access to a large fenced-in yard where Tara could run free. I was satisfied with my new situation, and I shared

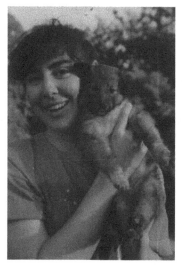

my good news with Zachary. He, in turn, told me he wanted to meet me in person, but our rendezvous would have to wait due to his work schedule. I hoped our burgeoning romance would turn into a genuine relationship, but a hunch told me my hopes would be in vain.

Smitten with Tara, my Sheltie puppy, Santa Cruz Mountains, California, 1991

CHAPTER SEVEN

A Glimpse of Bipolar

I drank my first cup of coffee when I was twenty-two years old. The momentous event occurred when I was the office manager of Silicon Events, a special event production company. I had been used to part-time jobs, and it was a shock to work a long stretch of tense, busy hours five days a week. I was slow to get going when we opened at 8:00 a.m., but after I drank my first cup of French Roast, I experienced a caffeine buzz. I welcomed the energy rush! I finally understood why the Kelly's French Pastries customers fussed over their to-go cups of the tasty brew. I was glad that the coffee machine was located a few feet away from my desk.

Silicon Events' skeleton crew of four staff required each of us to do a variety of duties. The lion's share of my job included office tasks such as accounting, filing, and answering phones. As time went on, my responsibilities became more interesting and challenging, especially when I worked at our summer events. I assisted Colin, the company's dark-haired, stocky founder, and his wife Sheryl, the creative director. Sheryl was a pretty, olive-skinned blonde with large, expressive brown eyes. The couple hired a development coordinator named Blake, a tall surfer and an atypically driven perfectionist who rounded out our team. Our Santa Cruz office was a three-hundred-square-foot room, and its lack of privacy was reminiscent of my airless UCSC converted lounge. None of us had cubicles, so we could overhear one another's phone conversations—it was a recipe for frustration. Sound barriers would have helped, but the room would have been more claustrophobic. Each of us got used to blocking out the others' voices, and Colin was often out of the office, which gave us one less distraction.

Silicon Events produced upscale, weekend music festivals that featured world-famous-musicians. Each event attracted hundreds of thousands of attendees. Colin had developed an outstanding reputation as a concert producer. After Colin had founded his company in affluent Silicon Valley, he brought Sheryl on board, and their talents complemented one another.

This was my first experience working for a perfectionist. When I answered the phone, I never knew what to expect. The caller could be a talent agent who represented Ray Charles or Etta James, or it could be a mellow Santa Cruz shaved ice vendor who hoped to rent a food booth at our next festival. None of them knew we worked out of an office not much bigger than a closet. Colin wanted his staff to give the level of sophisticated service talent agents would receive from a first-rate Los Angeles or New York-based company. If I made a mistake during a conversation, he'd overhear my faux pas. The moment I hung up the phone, Colin corrected me in a gruff voice. At least he didn't yell, but I felt humiliated and stupid all the same. I got the gist of the policies as quickly as I could.

I loved working with Sheryl, who was funny and caring. She complimented my work and appreciated my dedication. Sheryl's faith in my abilities boosted my confidence, and I was grateful to have her as my mentor. My witty co-worker Blake was two years older than me and acted like my protective brother. Blake was always willing to help me with a work project if I hit a snag. He was easy to work with, and we joked around often. Blake and I thrived in our first "grown-up" jobs, and we operated as a family more than as a business model. There was dysfunction among us, as there is with any family, but due to Colin and Sheryl's recognition of the importance of my role, I worked at their company for four years.

At Silicon Events, I established rapport with a range of professionals such as government agency representatives and media contacts. I worked with hundreds of food, art, and craft vendors who participated in the annual summer festivals we produced. I proudly considered myself a team player. However, at the start of every workday, a thick depression would hit me hard. I'd sit in my Jetta in the office complex parking lot. I dreaded the moment I'd have to force myself to walk to the office and don a fake smile. As anyone could imagine, it was exhausting to live that way. I was relieved no one ever questioned me about my mood. I worried if I revealed how bad I felt, I'd lose my job. I didn't confide in friends or family nor did I seek counseling, which would have been immensely helpful. My only outlet was writing in my journals.

When I sat down in my chair and drank a few cups of coffee, I could ignore my depression. Being busy the moment I walked in the door helped me to stop ruminating about how terrible I felt. I answered the phones in as much of an upbeat tone as I could. I returned home each night to Tara, my journal, and an empty studio, pessimistic and lonely.

During my time working for Silicon Events, I had symptoms of bipolar disorder briefly emerge. The bubbling over of my mood took place during the height of summer. We had spent months getting ready to produce a large Fourth of July festival that would be attended by thousands of people. It was my first time being in charge of handling logistics for twenty-five food vendors and seventy arts and crafts vendors. Vendor coordination is a formidable responsibility for anyone, especially someone like me who was new to event production.

On the eve of the festival, I stayed up all night to mark all the vendors' 10x10-foot booth spaces with chalk. I wanted to make sure everything was organized. I felt tremendous pressure to do an outstanding job. My sudden, extreme sleep deprivation triggered hypomania, and the next day I was hopped up. I had pressurized speech, racing thoughts, excessive energy, and irritability— all classic symptoms of mania. As my brain was on the verge of spiraling out of control, somehow I was able to handle my vendor responsibilities. My unusually gregarious personality made me a hit among the vendors, and I loved hearing them tell me how I was doing a standout job. Then an incident occurred that made it obvious to others that something was amiss with my brain.

I raced around the San Jose festival grounds holding my walkie-talkie. I was constantly fixing vendor-related dilemmas. One food vendor didn't like his arrogant neighbor, so I served as their peacemaker. A craft vendor asked me to help her move a heavy display. And so it went. I was treated like a queen by practically everyone, which only ramped up my exuberant state and feelings of grandiosity. The food vendors fed me their delectable specialty items throughout the day, and I was given free drinks and desserts that represented the diverse community of Silicon Valley's biggest city. Many craft vendors gifted me with their wares including jewelry, clothing—even a seventy-dollar hanging Sky Chair! The boost to my ego and the sugar in my system made me more hyper by the hour.

I thought my job was difficult until I observed Colin in action. I marveled at how he handled a ton of responsibilities so calmly. Anyone could tell he was dedicated to putting on a first-rate production. I was proud to be associated with his company.

That afternoon I walked through a shady grove and noticed a middle-aged woman who stood a foot away from Colin. She was yelling at him, and it was apparent she didn't know she was raging at the festival director. From where I stood, I couldn't understand what she was saying. As I moved closer to Colin to provide backup support, I noticed he listened patiently to her nonsensical rant. I should have followed his lead, but I felt something strange activate within me. While I had always been a non-confrontational person, I felt compelled to put this woman in her place. I strode up to Colin's side and glared at the woman's tomato-red face.

"Do you have *ANY* idea who this man is?" I shouted at her. I couldn't stop myself from unleashing my fury upon this stranger.

I continued hollering, "How dare you yell at him! He's the Festival Director!"

I moved closer to her, bulging my eyes so that I resembled the *Young Frankenstein* actor Marty Feldman. She might have sensed I was only getting started with my tirade, for she stopped yelling. Colin wanted the scene to end.

He glanced at my sweaty, livid face and said quietly, "Dyane, go take a break. It's okay."

Although my brain had gone haywire, I wasn't completely out of touch with reality. I knew Colin was curious about his introverted office manager's bizarre explosion, but he was wanted at the main music stage to deal with a logistical snafu. I had quickly gotten over my tantrum and had no remorse. I flitted about the festival grounds in an electric golf cart I had rented for the staff. Mania had dominated my cautious nature, and the high wasn't subsiding.

That same day, a woman approached me who was interested in being a last-minute arts and crafts vendor. We didn't accept last-minute vendors, but after I looked at her portfolio, I impulsively gave her a vacant space. In my manic state, I ignored our strict jurying process. My decision to break the rule was highly unethical, and it was unlike my normal behavior.

What I did next was worse.

After the vendor had paid me her booth fee in cash, I shoved the money in my pocket. When the day came to a close, I was overly giddy. My mania was still going strong, and I kept the vendor's money instead of depositing it into the festival's coffers. I spent the entire amount at various craft booths within fifteen minutes. My gleeful, obnoxious shopping spree was a spectacle. Some vendors were miffed I didn't spend money at their booths. Onlookers laughed at me when I walked by with my arms chock-full of beautiful clothes, jewelry, and other items. I had transformed myself into a walking clothes display rack.

Despite my extreme behavior, no one told me I might have a mood disorder. I could have lost my job when I broke festival rules, but I didn't think about the consequences. I was risk-taking, a classic symptom of mania, but I was clueless I had jeopardized my position with Silicon Events. I was unaware I damaged my integrity as a vendor coordinator. Because I wasn't held accountable for my behavior, I didn't perceive I had a problem.

The next two nights my extreme exhaustion caused me to resume my normal sleeping schedule. My mania abated, but my brain chemistry had been thrown totally askew. Like a dormant volcano, my bipolar disorder would eventually erupt in full force.

CHAPTER EIGHT

Settling for Less, Take Two

After the hectic festival season had ended, I scheduled a short vacation to meet Zachary. I was a bundle of nerves, yet filled with excitement. Everyone who learned about the circumstances in which we met was dubious about our relationship's future except for one person: Sheryl. A die-hard romantic, Sheryl was optimistic, and she used our coffee breaks to speculate about what Zachary would be like in person. On the other hand, my parents were less than thrilled I had a long-distance boyfriend.

As I drove ninety minutes to San Francisco International Airport to pick up Zachary, my palms left sweaty marks all over the steering wheel. *What am I getting myself into here?* I thought. *This is crazy!* I stood at the gate waiting for Zachary's plane to land, silently cursing myself for being so desperate I had to import a boyfriend.

I recognized Zachary from a picture he had sent me. Close to six feet tall, he was slim with wavy black hair, large brown eyes, and pale skin, and he stood out amongst the tanned, wiry California surfers that milled around us. He seemed sweet, but I didn't experience love at first sight.

I booked Zachary into a motel, and I gave him a tour of my adopted hometown. When he met Patricia, who had also grown up in New Jersey, they hit it off. I soaked up Zachary's attention, but it was a passionless connection. I swatted away the persistent thought that pursuing our relationship would be an enormous mistake. Soon after Zachary returned to New Jersey, he called me one night.

"I'd love to move to Santa Cruz," he said in his personable New Jersey accent.

"Okay," I replied as my stomach churned in protest. Thoughts such as *It's not the greatest idea to move in with a stranger!* and *You're not attracted to each other! You want a boyfriend, not a buddy!* came to mind, but I ignored them. I couldn't bear to be alone any longer. What I didn't realize was that living with someone else would be far lonelier than being by myself.

I obtained Patricia's permission for Zachary to move in, and the details fell into place. I brought Tara to Happy Tails Pet Boarding before I flew to New Jersey to meet Zachary's family. After staying in New Jersey for the weekend, we had planned to drive his car to Santa Cruz. It was an ambitious undertaking for any couple, let alone two people who barely knew each other.

My flight to Newark Airport was smooth, and a friendly seatmate distracted me by telling me about her travels. Zachary picked me up, and we drove to Cape May to meet his large family. Beautiful Victorian buildings dotted the peninsula that was surrounded by the magnificent Atlantic Ocean. It was a popular seaside tourist destination just like Santa Cruz, but I missed California and I was homesick. During my visit with his parents and seven brothers and sisters, I felt scrutinized, and my shyness came to the fore.

I watched Zachary interact with his family; they all adored him. I was the villain who was making off with their precious son and sibling. Out of eight children, Zachary was the only one who was moving out of state. I admired Zachary for his courage in making such a brave step. However, since I was considered responsible for luring him to the West Coast, it didn't feel good to be the pariah. I had expected that out of everyone, Zachary's mother would hold me most in contempt, but she was wonderful. She treated me like a friend, and her kindness helped me get through the visit.

Zachary stood out among his brothers and sisters as musically gifted, creative and intellectual. Encouraged to become a police officer rather than a university student, Zachary was bored, and desired a change in his life. He knew he'd have more opportunities to explore his talents in Santa Cruz's eclectic music scene instead of his conservative hometown. When the day arrived for us to make the long trek to California, we took turns driving Zachary's jam-packed Toyota Tercel over three thousand miles. Driving nonstop, we completed the cross-country route in only two and a half days.

Our relationship was doomed from the start. Despite my being a sensual, affectionate young woman, our pairing was devoid of any physical contact except for hugs. We treated each other as brother and sister, and I resigned myself to a dispassionate relationship. On weekends we explored the Santa Cruz restaurant scene and went to movies. He spent his spare time playing his guitar and composing songs while I read books and played with Tara. I helped Zachary find a job at a manufacturing company where his amiable personality fit in well with his coworkers. Although he made friends at work, he was essentially a loner.

On a breezy Saturday afternoon, I spotted my West Cliff Drive housemate Mark walking a puppy down my street. I flagged down Mark, and he introduced me to Paco. The puppy looked like a giant cotton ball with bright black eyes. When I crouched down to pet him, I flashed back to the days when Tara was a puppy. Mark said Paco was an American Eskimo, a highly intelligent breed used for circus performers. I was amazed to learn the spunky canines could dance to music, perform with clowns, walk on wires, and weave in and out of wagon wheels!

Although Mark lived three blocks from my studio, I hadn't seen him in some time. At our last get-together, he'd told me how lonely he felt. I was glad to see Mark with this loving, fun companion.

"Where did you find Paco?" I asked.

"Oh, I got him from my Uncle Jim in Florida," Mark replied.

"Does your uncle have any more puppies?" I asked him with a grin.

"How about I get in touch with him, and I'll find out!" he said.

A few days later Mark called and said his uncle was planning to visit Santa Cruz in a few weeks. I impulsively arranged for Uncle Jim to bring me an American Eskimo puppy. I set everything in motion without consulting Zachary or Patricia. In the past, I did nothing to jeopardize my lease with a landlord, but my frustration over my unfulfilling platonic relationship had affected my decision-making. Zachary took my puppy plan in stride, but he was concerned that Patricia would be furious and ask us to leave.

I met Uncle Jim at the San Francisco Airport, and we went to collect my puppy in her crate. I named her Shera after the cartoon character in the 1980s kids' television show *He-Man and She-Ra*. I should have researched the American Eskimo temperament with other breeds, but I assumed if I introduced a puppy to Tara, they'd have a good chance at getting along.

I knew I made a mistake by not communicating with Zachary and Patricia. I was prepared to apologize to Patricia so we'd have a chance of remaining in her studio, but even if I groveled to her, she could still evict us. It was too late to do anything but hope she'd show us mercy. Patricia was angry I had brought Shera home without asking permission, but she only scolded me for a few minutes and didn't mention eviction. When our meeting ended, I sprinted for the studio so I could bask in the unconditional love of my canine family.

Zachary and I lived together for two more years. He made no romantic gestures, and I followed his lead. Our lackluster dynamic further contributed to my chronic depression. The disheartening situation resembled what I had with Eric. Once again I was unhappy, but I didn't have the self-confidence to leave an unfulfilling, unhealthy relationship.

When Zachary's childhood friend Lisa started calling him every evening from her New Jersey home, I crumbled. He took her calls in the bathroom so I didn't hear a word. Zachary told me Lisa was getting divorced, and she needed a friend's shoulder to cry on.

"Let her find another damn friend!" I yelled.

Zachary's willingness to be Lisa's confidante made me insecure and jealous. He denied he was in love with Lisa, but I intuitively knew he had romantic feelings for her. Although Lisa lived thousands of miles away, Zachary and I knew how relationships could be kindled through phone calls. Soon after Lisa entered our lives, Zachary acted strangely. He stopped sleeping. He talked in a strange, affected voice. He bought a bunch of white Hanes T-shirts to use as canvases for bizarre, intricate illustrations that he drew with black Sharpie pens. Then, without telling me or anyone else beforehand, he shaved off all his hair.

A few days after Zachary shaved his head, he told me he wanted out of our relationship. He confirmed my suspicions and announced he had fallen in love with Lisa. Even though he wasn't behaving like himself, I was humiliated at his rejection, and my terror reemerged at the prospect of being left alone. The awful situation caused my energy to dwindle, and I became listless. After Zachary had informed me he was leaving, he packed his possessions into his car and disappeared. I called in sick to Silicon Events. I couldn't get out of bed except to go to the bathroom, feed the dogs, and let them outside for a few minutes. I felt as if a giant boulder had pinned me down and I had no strength to move. After doing any task that required me to stand, I returned to bed spent.

I made a brief phone call to my parents to let them know about the break-up. They had been praying I'd move on from the relationship as soon as possible. These were the days before Skype and FaceTime, and my mother and father couldn't see my pallid, tearful face. They didn't realize how bad my mental state was because I deliberately kept my depression from them. I didn't have the energy or willingness to be interrogated about my dismal mood.

Another day passed, and I couldn't get out of bed for longer than a few minutes to feed the dogs and let them outside. Sheryl called, and I told her Zachary had broken up with me, but I didn't mention returning to work. I couldn't imagine ever going back to Silicon Events the way I was feeling.

"Oh Dyane, I'm so sorry," Sheryl said. "Take time off and let us know if we can do anything to help. You've accrued vacation days, so don't worry about work. Cathy can cover for you—that's the beauty of having an intern. Let's touch base next week," she said with extra warmth in her voice. Tears spilled down my cheeks as I listened to her.

My mother called my godmother Sarah, who was living abroad, and let her know about my break-up. Sarah called me as soon as she could, and as a former therapist, she could tell my depression was severe. She implored me to see a Santa Cruz psychiatrist she knew named Dr. Clark. Sarah assured me he was down-to-earth, and she guaranteed that it would be worth the effort to meet with him. I had never spent time with a psychiatrist except for the ones who milled around my father during his UCLA hospitalizations. I was feeling worse, and speaking with Sarah convinced me to see the psychiatrist. It comforted me to have a personal referral. I fervently hoped Dr. Clark could help me return to life. I took an extended leave of absence from my job and made an appointment.

CHAPTER NINE

Welcome to Psychiatry

Shera and Tara, the innocent victims of my depression, sat by my bed day after day and gained weight from their lack of activity. The studio smelled fetid from my unwashed body. With my desperation at an all-time high, I gathered every ounce of strength I had to drive fifteen minutes to Dr. Clark's office.

Dr. Clark, a tall, robust man in his late fifties, set me at ease with his warm greeting. He asked me basic medical history questions in a soothing voice. I leaned back into a comfortable leather chair and glanced at my surroundings. The psychiatrist's office looked like a cozy living room. Having my godmother's personal referral reduced my anxiety a little, but it was incredibly tough to meet with a stranger when I felt so despondent.

It was difficult focusing on Dr. Clark's words. My thought process had slowed down, and I couldn't comprehend his explanation about depression. Dr. Clark noted my lack of expression and switched gears to avoid overwhelming me. He was aware my father had bipolar disorder, but I didn't show up with manic symptoms and I didn't mention my manic Silicon Events weekend. After talking with me for almost an hour, Dr. Clark diagnosed me with clinical depression.

He prescribed paroxetine, an antidepressant in the selective serotonin reuptake inhibitor (SSRI) group. At age twenty-five, paroxetine was my first psychiatric medication. Dr. Clark wound down our session by explaining the importance of regulating my circadian rhythm. He defined circadian as regular twenty-four-hour-long cycles and he encouraged me to stop sleeping all the time, a typical symptom of clinical depression. "Make sure you get up during the daytime every day!" he insisted.

Dr. Clark urged me to get outdoors and do some form of daily exercise. He suggested I walk around my neighborhood. It was the most feasible idea because Tara and Shera needed walks, particularly after being so sedentary. I picked up paroxetine at the pharmacy, timing the visit so that few shoppers would be there. I was embarrassed to interact with anyone because of my depression. I took the dogs for a walk that afternoon, and gradually increased our time from ten minutes to an hour. I began slowly pulling out of the deep hole of depression, but the intense feelings of hopelessness, loneliness, and purposelessness continued to plague me.

At the same time I struggled with clinical depression, Zachary suffered a mental crisis. After he had broken up with me, he rented a studio in a neighborhood that was notorious for drug dealing. One day his older brother John called me about Zachary's worsening mental condition. He mentioned Zachary's friend Lisa had moved three hours north of Santa Cruz to live with her aunt. Zachary had driven to Lisa's aunt's home, and his strange appearance disturbed her so much that the aunt filed a restraining order against him.

John called me again a few days later, and I learned Zachary had been hospitalized in a psychiatric unit near San Francisco. Although we were no longer together, I felt sorry for him. John wanted to help his brother, and he told me he'd visit Zachary as soon as he could take leave from his police officer job. Since John wouldn't arrive for several weeks, I decided to visit Zachary at the hospital. I had made substantial progress in my recovery to be able to make such a trip. Our meeting was brief, and Zachary was forlorn and heavily medicated. Later on, John called to tell me how much he and the rest of his family appreciated my visiting Zachary in light of what had happened between us. He wasn't aware of my depression, and I wasn't planning on telling him. I was deeply ashamed of having depression, and from past conversations with Zachary I knew that John and the rest of his family looked down upon any mental illness, even when it came to their beloved Zachary.

When Zachary was discharged from the hospital, he returned to Santa Cruz only to relapse again. John, now in Santa Cruz, left me a message saying Zachary was admitted to the local Behavioral Health Unit, a short drive from my studio. I called Zachary to ask if I could visit him, but he declined.

"I don't want you to see this place, Dyane," he insisted. "It's horrible—there are people shitting on themselves right in front of me!" I didn't want to aggravate him and I respected his request. Moreover, I was glad to be off the hook. Zachary's description of the place frightened me. I could only imagine he was in some kind of hellhole.

It was beyond my wildest dreams I'd end up in the same psychiatric unit a decade later.

Zachary's family would eventually tell me that when he was a teenager, he had a psychotic break and spent a month in a psychiatric hospital. I wasn't given any other details, so I don't know if he was given a bipolar disorder diagnosis. My ignorance of his mental health history did Zachary a great disservice. If I had known details about his first hospitalization, I could have watched for signs of relapse. The fact that he and his family didn't inform me about his hospitalization before he moved to California was indicative of the stigma associated with mental illness.

As Zachary began taking medication, he became stable and returned to work. I pulled back from interacting with him. I had focused on his illness and its accompanying drama, in part, to distract me from my mental health issues. Fortunately, I realized I had to move on.

I took Tara and Shera for walks at Lighthouse Field State Park. Walking briskly for an hour had become effortless. I looked forward to taking in the breathtaking view of the crashing Pacific Ocean. The dogs enthusiastically explored the field and played well with most of the other dogs we encountered. As I learned how to manage my depression, I grew stronger mentally. I remained on paroxetine and decided not to return to my high-pressured Silicon Events job. I did the necessary paperwork for temporary disability income and occasionally received small checks from my parents.

Although I loved my park excursions, the weather became rainy and cold. I took the dogs out for shorter walks, but I wanted an indoor place to exercise. A new gym named Banana Slug Fitness was opening downtown and they advertised a low introductory rate. The owners were an upbeat, attractive French couple named Roland and Manon. They believed that fitness should not only be effective but fun. I was drawn to their philosophy, and I liked supporting a family-owned, local business. I bought a year's membership and rationalized the expense as an investment in my mental health. The membership included three sessions with a certified personal trainer. I paid close attention to the trainer's techniques, and because I had plenty of free time, my muscles grew strong. Physically, I had improved a vast amount since my bedridden days. While I was doing better mentally, I was still fragile.

Feeling lost without a job to give me purpose and a routine, I started imagining myself as a certified personal trainer. I thought it would be fulfilling to help people learn how to be healthier. My Palisades YMCA and Banana Slug Fitness experiences had made me a believer in the power of weight training. As I contemplated becoming a trainer, I started looking for a new place to live. My studio held too many upsetting memories of Zachary and my depression. It was time for a new start.

CHAPTER TEN

Starting Over

Isn't it nice to think that tomorrow is a new day with no mistakes in it yet?

L.M. Montgomery, *Anne of Green Gables*

Studio hunting had become a familiar, tedious routine. Each morning I scanned the newspaper's classified section for studio rentals. I wanted a studio so I could hide my depression from others. Studios had become rare, and I only found shared housing vacancies. I noticed an advertisement for a room rental in my neighborhood that fit my budget. Taking a deep breath, I dialed the phone number. After a few rings, a man answered. My first question would determine whether we would speak further.

"Hi! My name is Dyane. I'm calling about the room for rent. Do you consider dogs?" I asked.

"Hi, I'm Steven. Dogs are fine—as long as they aren't like Cujo," he said. "I have a dog named Timothy. He's old and blind, but he's pretty good with other dogs. I bet he'd like some company because I'm the only one living here. I have to warn you— I'm a computer nerd."

"That's fine. You could be something *much* worse!" I said. Steven paused, then roared with laughter.

We agreed to meet in the late afternoon. Steven greeted me sporting a thick black braid that reached to his waist. It was a bold look for a computer nerd, and I liked his originality. We spoke for a while in the living room, and he told me about his job as a computer engineer. The elderly Timothy meandered around the living room, oblivious to Shera and Tara. We went to explore the large, grassy yard, and the dogs made themselves at home. The vacant room was shabby-but-livable.

Steven's easygoing manner won me over, and I wanted the room. The phone rang several times while I was there. From the sound of Steven's brief conversations, there were other applicants vying for the rental. I needed to stand out among the competition, and I knew what could give me the upper hand. I stopped by Emily's, a popular Westside bakery, and bought a luscious dark chocolate cake. I delivered the treat to Steven with a note saying how much I'd like to live there. Steven called late that evening to ask when I could move in.

After I settled into my new home, I had enough motivation to pursue working at the gym. Since I had no experience as a fitness trainer, I thought I'd apply for a front desk reception position. I figured reception had to be a far less stressful job than special event production. I told a staff member about my interest in employment at the gym. She said she was moving away soon, and her reception job would be available. It was the perfect time to ask for an application form, and I pounced on the opportunity.

During my interview with Roland, I was nervous and silently chastised myself for feeling and acting so shaky. In spite of my anxiety, I made a positive impression on him, and he hired me to work the morning shift five days a week. Roland warned me it would be challenging to wake up early and greet members warmly at the crack of dawn. In a charming French accent, he explained how much he wanted Banana Slug Fitness to stand apart from the other gyms. He joked that even though the French had a reputation for being rude, he believed in friendly, sincere customer service. I wondered if I could meet his high expectations. I recalled the phrase "Fake it 'til you make it" and I knew that's what I had to do.

On my first day of work at Banana Slug Fitness, I woke up at the dark, chilly hour of 4:45 a.m. to shower before my shift. The hot water helped wake me up, and when I was clean, I felt more confident. I arrived at the gym at 5:30 and followed a list of opening duties. At 6:00 a.m. I unlocked the entrance, checked in the early bird members, and gave them workout towels. I made an effort to be friendly to everyone, and when Roland said I was one of the members' favorite employees, I was thrilled. Not everything went so well. I struggled the most when I asked members to pay their past-due bills, and I wasn't wild about cleaning the men's bathroom.

My depression was kept at bay by my job routine and the exercise I did at the gym after my shift. I took on more responsibility, and my self-esteem was on the mend. The head trainer knew I was interested in a fitness career. He said I'd need to become a certified trainer to work at any credible gym. I took the plunge and charged the expensive study materials for the American Council on Exercise (A.C.E.) personal training certification on my credit card. I committed myself to study every day. I wasn't dating, I had few friends, and I didn't see Steven much at home, but I was grateful to get out of bed, interact with the world, and have a goal.

I had no educational background in anatomy, physiology, or the latest exercise research. I was overwhelmed by the massive amount of information in the A.C.E. course guide. The book was so heavy I could have used it to do bicep curls! I did my best learning in a classroom with a teacher, but there were no A.C.E. classes available in my area. I made flash cards and took sample tests. I found the material as difficult as any class I took in college. When I visualized working as an A.C.E. trainer, I felt good about taking on a new identity. I wouldn't want to work in a gym forever, but I thought being a certified trainer would be a useful skill.

Several months later, I drove up to the San Francisco-based high school where A.C.E. was administering the test. I was an apprehensive jangle of nerves. If I didn't pass, I could re-take the exam at a hefty price, but I had studied so hard, and I wanted to do well. Roland, Manon, and all of my other coworkers knew I was testing for my certification, and the last thing I wanted to do was tell them I failed. My hands were freezing and sticky as I grabbed my pencil and filled in several hundred bubbles on the Scantron form. Three hours later our time was up, and I was exhausted. I drove at a snail's pace back home as I reflected on some of the most baffling questions such as "What's the difference between anabolism vs. catabolism?" and "What's the Karvonen formula?" There was a strong chance that I blew it, and I was upset the rest of the day. Unlike today's immediate test result notification technology, in the late 1990s, it took four weeks to receive the test results. Every afternoon I checked the mail hoping for an envelope filled with good news. At last, our mail carrier delivered a slim form that would indicate if my four-hundred-dollar test fee had been paid in vain. I ripped it open to see I had *barely* passed, but I did it! I burst into tears. I was relieved and proud I had accomplished my goal all on my own.

Although my self-worth increased after passing the A.C.E. exam, I was single, and I didn't have my eye on anyone. When I observed loving couples at the gym, my heart would squeeze with loneliness. As much as I didn't want to admit it, depression was not only lurking, it was intensifying. I was experiencing *dysthymia*, a serious, chronic state of depression that can last up to two years. Dysthymia is classified in the *Diagnostic and Statistical Manual of Mental Disorders (DSM-5)* as *persistent depressive disorder*. I was no longer taking paroxetine or seeing Dr. Clark. I exercised, ate healthy food, and got enough sleep, but I was in despair. I didn't seek professional help again because my depression had clouded my mind, and all logic went out the window. I didn't realize that appropriate treatment could have helped me feel much better. No one told me I had a problem, and I continued to neglect my mental health.

I was adept at hiding my feelings at the gym's front counter. I put on a good show while I interacted with high-powered members including the Editor-in-Chief of the *Santa Cruz Sentinel*, the Executive Director of the Santa Cruz Museum of Art, and the co-founder of Netflix. Working at the front desk gave me the chance to socialize with members, and some of them knew I was college educated. The members who were aware of my UCSC background treated me with respect—I wasn't merely the "counter girl."

The only person I saw fairly often was Craig, Steve's best friend. Craig was a tall blonde geologist who had met Steve in a scuba diving class. When we were introduced, I liked him straight away, but I was only interested in friendship. My depression had tamped down my ability to feel attracted to anyone.

One day Steven asked me, "What do you think of Craig?"

"Oh, he isn't my type!" I said.

Craig and Steven spent much of their free time at the house while I holed myself up in my room. Craig knew I was struggling, and he did thoughtful things for me. He fixed my guitar. He paid attention to my dogs and played with them in the backyard. If Craig cooked something for himself and Steven, he'd offer me a plate of food. I was self-absorbed, another side effect of depression, and I never gave Craig anything but a wan smile for his graciousness.

Life stopped being routine when Granny was diagnosed with lung cancer. As soon as I heard the news over the phone from my mother, I started sobbing. Granny declined rapidly. The last time I saw her was at Santa Monica's St. John's Hospital, and she didn't recognize me. Granny was in such distress she screamed at me for no reason—it was the first time she had ever raised her voice at me. As tears streamed down my face, I panicked and sprinted out of the room. I felt cowardly and guilty, but I wasn't strong enough to deal with her agony.

After I returned to Santa Cruz, my mother moved Granny back to her apartment for hospice care. Granny's death increased my dysthymic depression twofold, and I felt like I was walking through a mudslide. I should have hightailed it back to Dr. Clark and gotten medication to see me through the aftermath of Granny's death, but I told no one about how terrible I felt. Roland and Manon were compassionate and supportive, and said my family came first. They gave me two weeks of paid time off and a sympathy card. They knew how much I loved my Granny. Steven and Craig offered to care for my dogs, and I flew to New York with my family for Granny's funeral.

Granny was buried next to her mother Esther at a cemetery in upstate New York. Her prize pupil Congressman Charles Rangel attended her memorial. She had been so proud of Congressman Rangel, the first African-American Chair of the United States House Ways and Means Committee. In a minor miracle, I brought a miniature tape recorder so I could record his heartfelt eulogy. I wanted to listen to it someday when my grief didn't control my every thought.

When I returned to work at Banana Slug Fitness, my depression had lightened enough for me to put on my "mask." I smiled at work, but I felt hollow inside. My workouts helped improve my mood a little, as did being in familiar surroundings, but I hated feeling so cheerless. I was sick of seeing lovey-dovey members hold hands as they walked through the door—I was more than sick of it; I was green with envy. The negative, hopeless voices in my brain droned: *You'll never find the love you want—who would want to be with the real you?*

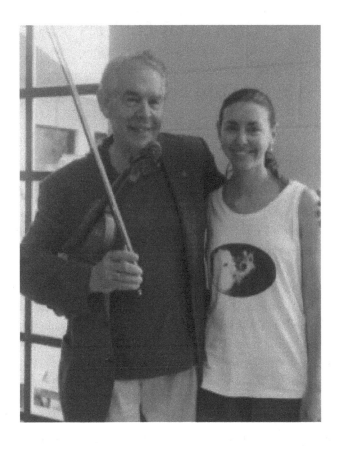

With my father at Banana Slug Fitness, Santa Cruz, California, 1997.

CHAPTER ELEVEN

When You Least Expect It

After Granny's death, I increased my workouts to see if the greater effort would lift my depression. I exercised for an hour after work, and never skipped a session unless I was sick. At the close of my Friday shift, Craig showed up unexpectedly. He was working from home and took a break to invite me to coffee. Until that day, I had abided by my rule to never play workout hooky. Spring was in the air, and I was getting a little burned out on my stringent routine. The world would not end if I skipped one workout. I impulsively broke my rule and told Craig I'd join him for espresso at LuLu Carpenter's Café. We had a mellow conversation in which I quizzed him about earthquakes and tsunamis. After an hour, I stood up to leave. Craig didn't give me our customary brief hug, but he kissed me lightly on the side of my neck. I was completely taken aback, and I couldn't help but laugh at the unusual gesture—it was a real laugh too, not my usual pretending act.

"Are you a vampire?" I asked.

"Of course not!" Craig sputtered.

After years of living without a shred of romance, it felt good to be desired.

The more I got to know Craig, the more I noticed his appealing attributes. He had a high-level job at a geological engineering company. He was outdoorsy, he liked to cook, and he was a talented guitarist. Ten years older than me, he was mature and grounded. A few days after our LuLu Carpenters chat, Craig asked me to a weekend brunch at the Davenport Cash Store. Over scrambled eggs and coffee, something had changed. I couldn't deny there was chemistry between us, and it was exciting! I was drawn to Craig, but I was scared that I'd become enmeshed in another disastrous relationship. My fear was irrational, but my failed relationships had made me paranoid.

The following week, Craig and a friend were going backpacking in the Sierras. A few hours before he left, I wrote him an email that jumped the gun and suggested we should only be friends. In an attempt to soften the blow of my message, I listed every quality I liked about him. As soon as I pressed the "send" key, I realized I had made a gigantic mistake. Ten minutes after I sent the email, I emailed Craig again and asked him if we could meet after he returned from the mountains.

Two days later, I received an email from Craig. He wrote,

"Dyane,

I just got back from the Sierras. I always get a little rush when I see a message from you. This one rather knocked the wind out of me.

The truth is, recently I've been kind of holding my breath because...I have been falling for you for a million reasons—reasons that seem totally natural. It seems like something has been going on with you too, but I've been in doubt because I've never seen myself as the kind of guy who can pull someone so desirable.

You are all the things you said about me (intelligent, sexy, etc.). The compliments are very flattering, but Dyane, to tell you the absolute truth, I'm just a guy who

wants to be loved and to love someone who I care about.
I seek someone who I can open up to emotionally and
trust...it's fundamental. But it sounds like you've made a
decision, so there's not much I can say or do.

I'm delirious from the trip, and I would like to talk
with you. Tomorrow night is fine.

Love,
Craig"

At the appointed time, I drove to Craig's apartment across the
street from the historic Santa Cruz Mission. I wondered if it was
too late to fix the mess I had created. I felt idiotic for giving him
mixed messages and for risking our chance to be together. When I
walked into his apartment, I couldn't say a word. Craig looked at
me, and I wrapped my arms around him in a big hug. The energy
between us was something I had never felt with anyone before.

I find the phrase "fall in love" apt. Although I'd never bungee
jump off a bridge, I bungee jumped in an emotional sense when
our relationship began. I was more than ready to take the plunge
if it meant being with Craig. I radiated happiness, and everyone I
encountered at the gym could tell a special person had come into
my life. Craig called his mother Marcia in Hawaii to tell her about
me, and I called my parents to gush about him. The people in our
lives had observed our loneliness for a long time, and they were
happy for us. I shared my history of depression with Craig, and he
knew about my father's bipolar disorder.

For the time being, I continued renting my room in Steven's
house. Craig gave me a key to his apartment and treated me so
lovingly that I thought our relationship was too good to be true.
We went on day-trips south to Big Sur, north to Pescadero, and
out to dinner at our favorite restaurants. I wasn't spending much
time with my dogs at the house, and I felt guilty. Steven gave them
lots of attention, but he worked long shifts. Craig suggested we

swap living spaces with Steven. The idea was perfect, for Steven had always envied Craig's downtown Santa Cruz apartment, and he agreed to the exchange.

Despite my newfound happiness, I was restless working at Banana Slug Fitness. I was tired of waking up so early each weekday, and while it was fulfilling to train members, I still had to do plenty of physical grunt work. I recalled a conversation I had with a member named Brian, the Executive Director of the Downtown Association. At six feet, four inches, Brian had a strapping build, and he was full of ambition. When I started working at the gym, I mentioned my background in special event production to him, and he had offered me a job interview on the spot. I declined as graciously as I could. Now I wanted to know if there might be a position available. I called Brian, and he invited me to interview for a development coordinator job. I was impressed with his connection to the Santa Cruz creative scene. I wanted to work in a place devoid of sweat, but as nice as the office was, something didn't feel right

After our interview, Brian called me with a job offer with a generous salary. My intuition told me to pass, but I ignored it and accepted the position. Craig was proud of me for landing the job, and he gave me plenty of encouragement. I was grateful to leave Banana Slug Fitness on excellent terms with Roland and Manon. They were sorry to see me go, but they told me they wanted what was best for me. Despite the intimidation of tackling a new job, I was excited about a career change. After wearing shorts, sweats, and gym t-shirts for more than two years, I needed office-appropriate pieces of clothing. I bought stylish outfits that were a far cry from my gym uniform. I had a private office that overlooked downtown Santa Cruz, and I decorated it with a framed Wyland dolphin poster I loved. I was introduced to Marie, the office manager. An attractive, dark-haired petite woman in her late forties, Marie welcomed me so warmly I thought we might become friends. Marie's cordiality and sense of humor made it a pleasure to come to work. Unfortunately, she wouldn't be cracking jokes around me for long.

Shortly after my job began, I was bored out of my skull. The Downtown Association's minuscule Antique Faire took place in a parking lot, and it was dull compared to Silicon Events' 4th of July Extravaganza. Apart from the Antique Faire, I wasn't given much to do. But then something happened that made a bad situation intolerable.

I was scheduled to take a professional headshot for the Downtown Association's brochure. Marie hadn't been asked to participate. Her job was behind-the-scenes, and Brian didn't think a photo of her was necessary. When she found out about my photo session, she flew into a rage.

"Why didn't I get to take a photo? It's not fair!" she yelled at Brian in the reception room as if she were a toddler having a tantrum. I made myself scarce and hid in my office. From that day on, whenever we were near one another, Marie acted jealous, rude, and immature. The office environment became a toxic one, and despite having Craig in my life, my severe depression surfaced.

Marie's atrocious behavior had pushed me over the brink, and I quit. My depression grew worse, and the familiar feelings of shame and hopelessness overtook me. I tried hiding my depression from Craig, but he knew something was wrong. He supported my decision to leave the Downtown Association, and I left a message on Dr. Clark's voicemail in the hopes I could meet with him and apply for temporary disability. Dr. Clark was on sabbatical in another part of the country, but he referred me to a new psychiatrist.

I forced myself to deliver my resignation in person. I walked into Brian's office wearing my standard depression uniform of sweats and a grubby t-shirt. I was the complete opposite of my business-suited self. Marie had been told I was coming in, and was nowhere in sight. I had no idea how Brian would take my news about my mental illness. I sat down across from him, unable to look at his face. Anxiety and shame clutched at my heart.

"Brian, I have a bad case of…of depression, and I won't be able to work here anymore. I'm sorry."

"Dyane, I'm the one who's sorry. I understand," he said contritely. "And I realize I made a big mistake regarding Marie's unprofessional behavior. I didn't handle it the way I should have. I know it's too late now, but I'm truly sorry."

When I heard the regret in his voice, I looked him in the eye. I didn't want to cry, but two fat tears welled up in my eyes. I appreciated his kindness and his apology, but the damage had been done; my depression wasn't going to magically disappear. I shook hands with Brian and left his office to gather my things. I threw my office supplies into a box, but I left my Wyland dolphin poster behind. It was sentimental, but my depression had caused anhedonia (an inability to feel pleasure) and it erased my love for precious things. I walked out of the Downtown Association, never to return.

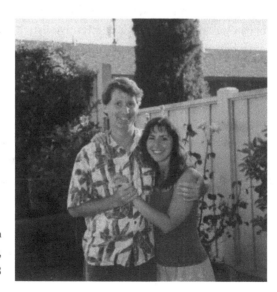

Happy times with Craig, Scotts Valley, California, 1998

CHAPTER TWELVE

Moments and Milestones

After my stint at the Downtown Association, I struggled to put one foot in front of the other. I learned how all the love in the world couldn't cure my chronic depression. Craig could only do so much to help me, and I couldn't stand being melancholy around him. I hoped with every fiber of my miserable soul that my appointment with my new psychiatrist Dr. Gordon would help me.

I drove to Dr. Gordon's office alone, unsure if I'd be able to do it, but I wanted to be less dependent on Craig. I was relieved when I arrived. Dr. Gordon was in his early sixties, tall and thin with neatly combed white hair. He was reserved, but once we began talking, he was a kind, attentive listener. I liked him. I met with him weekly and I took paroxetine again, which helped take me out of the doldrums.

As I pulled out of the depression, I wondered what to do to occupy myself. When I received my tax return refund, I registered for massage school. Ever since college, I loved indulging in professional massages to reduce stress. When I worked at the gym, I had considered taking a massage class to improve my anatomical knowledge, but I put the idea on hold. Now I had the money and the time to go for it. Passing the course would give me a sense of pride, and I could work as a massage therapist.

Santa Cruz was a massage-loving town with several schools to consider. Redwood Health Institute had a good reputation, and it was the most affordable option. Nervous and excited, I enrolled for the Wednesday night course. At the first class, Redwood's founder Pat Wellington explained his philosophy. He believed in the healing power of massage and he planned to teach us modalities I knew nothing about, such as polarity. When he introduced his co-teachers Diana and Perry, they smiled warmly at our group of twenty students.

After two weeks, my ambition to become a massage therapist fizzled. I had difficulties memorizing and executing the different moves. When I practiced techniques on my classmates, I was jittery and I shamefacedly dripped sweat on them. Our final exam was to give an instructor a massage, and it was scheduled after our dinner break. It was a warm evening, and I wore my usual outfit of an old tank top and sweats. Craig had mentioned he'd stop by for dinner so we could grab a quick bite to eat.

I hoped I'd avoid drowning my instructor with my perspiration and that somehow I'd miraculously pass the exam. Craig arrived after the lecture and suggested we visit Star Bene, a cozy Italian restaurant that overlooked the ocean. I hid my grungy clothes with a long coat and we were on our way.

We sat in the back courtyard at a small candlelit table and listened to the waves crashing softly. I wished I could stay at the restaurant for the rest of the evening rather than return to my dreaded exam. Glancing around at the attractively dressed diners, I was self-conscious my hair was coated with massage oil, but at least it was dark outside.

After we had ordered dinner, Craig pulled out a green velvet box and placed it on the table between us.

"Open it," he said in a low voice.

I opened the box to find a beautiful white gold, diamond, and sapphire engagement ring. It was dainty, and I loved the simple design. My jaw dropped—I did *not* expect this to happen on this particular night!

"Will you?" he asked me. I knew the rest...

"Yes!" I said.

A customer who had been watching us from indoors sprinted to our table.

"Did I see what I *think* I saw?" she belted out. Other patrons jerked their heads in our direction. We smiled, and nodded yes.

"Congratulations—how wonderful!" she exclaimed, and jogged back to her table.

I stared in awe at the sparkling ring on my finger. Craig mentioned it was time to return to the Redwood Health Institute. When I walked into my class, I was beaming and told everyone what had happened over dinner. I carefully took the ring off my finger and secured it in its case. When I began my exam with my teacher Diana, I suspect my happiness might have affected her more than my massage moves because after I finished, she announced I had passed!

After I had finished my course, I began planning our wedding. Craig was open to any idea as long as the costs were kept down. My engagement and daily exercise reduced my depression a great deal. I continued my sessions with Dr. Gordon and continued taking a low dose of paroxetine. I was preoccupied with the novelty of paging through wedding magazines, researching caterers, sampling chocolate cakes, scouting potential locations, and searching for the perfect dress. I set my sights on creating a unique, meaningful celebration.

October was my favorite time of year, and Craig and I agreed that fall in the Santa Cruz Mountains would be the perfect time to get married. We knew of an ideal place to hold our ceremony: Quail Hollow Ranch, a county park popular with hikers and birders. Quail Hollow was the former residence of *Sunset* magazine publisher Laurence W. Lane. The park was also home to the Santa Cruz Sandhills, a habitat of plants and animals found nowhere else on earth! The three-hundred-acre nature preserve's rental fee was low because it was county-park-owned.

Although I confirmed most of the logistics, I grew more and more anxious. Some brides love being the center of attention, but I wasn't looking forward to it. I was nervous about meeting Craig's mother and sister. I desperately wanted to make a good impression upon them, but I felt certain I'd make a fool of myself. Years of grappling with low self-esteem and a poor body image had taken a toll on me, and my emotional phantoms were flaring up.

In an attempt to settle my nerves, I worked out compulsively at Banana Slug Fitness. For the first time in my life, I was too thin. At least the consistent exercise helped keep my depression in check and getting married gave me a positive focus. But soon an unimaginable tragedy would affect us all.

It was the year 2001. Three weeks before our wedding day, the horrific terrorist attacks of 9/11 took place. Many of us watched the media coverage, unable to look away from images destined to give us nightmares for years to come. The terrorist attacks of 9/11 activated my father's bipolar depression, which was one of the worst depressions he ever had. During a phone conversation, he told me he didn't think he could make it to our wedding. I couldn't imagine my father missing our ceremony. Dad's condition shook me to the core, and my anxiety skyrocketed. My mother and brother assured me that he would attend our ceremony. I didn't want to admit it, but I was angry with my father. I should have been compassionate, but I was on edge.

As the case has been for scores of brides and grooms, our wedding day was a blur. I barely slept the night before the ceremony. This sudden lack of sleep would explain my erratic behavior over the next twenty-four hours.

One of our wedding's highlights was the participation of our dogs. Tara was our flower girl, bedecked with a corsage of flame-colored calla lilies. Shera's fluffy white fur matched the color of my wedding dress. She joined us for dancing after the ceremony, gleefully darting in between our guests on the brick patio. There were mishaps galore. Our sweet caterer Erika smashed the historic house's window while carrying a tray. Luckily she was unharmed, although her paycheck took a hit to cover the window's repair. The day's weather forecast had been sunny and warm, but it turned out to be foggy, cold, and dismal. No one touched the pitchers of ice water on the tables. The bridesmaids wore sweatpants underneath their dresses to keep warm, but I was hot from all the excitement.

The biggest mistake I made in planning our wedding was choosing our officiant. I hired Redwood Health Institute's Pat Wellington. He had been such a charismatic speaker and Craig liked his style too. I assumed Pat charged the going rate of one hundred dollars. However, his contract listed a five-hundred-dollar fee. Too intimidated to counteroffer, I agreed to the ridiculously high amount. My parents offered to pay his bill as our wedding gift, and while they grumbled about the cost, they said the choice was up to us.

On our wedding day when Pat read the ceremony script I had written, it was clear he had not read it closely beforehand. He made so many mistakes I wondered if he was drunk. He paused excessively, slurred his words, and swayed. He had never done any of those behaviors during his massage lectures. To top it off, he forgot to introduce Sharon, our maid of honor, who was performing Carole King's song "Way Over Yonder." He didn't have us sign the marriage license, which I didn't think was a major problem, but that oversight would prove to cause me enormous stress later on. My mother gave him a substantial pay cut, and he didn't contest it. Our dogs would've done a better job of performing the marriage ceremony.

My disappointment with Pat paled in comparison to the most difficult part of the day: seeing my father in such a depressed state. When we joined arms to walk to the podium, he shuffled slowly and didn't seem present. After Dad released my arm to take his seat, he looked confused and stood there for a long, awkward moment. I was unsure if he could make the ten-foot walk to his table by himself, but he made it.

I didn't eat a mouthful of Erika's succulent dinner of organic chicken, maple-roasted sweet potatoes, and wild rice. I didn't have a bite of Black China Bakery's magnificent vegan chocolate cake that made our guests swoon. Erika had packed two boxes of food for us to take when we left the ranch, but Craig and I were so flustered, we forgot our meals. Thus, my only "meal" for the occasion was alcohol. I drank too much Perrier Jouët champagne before, during, and after the ceremony. That evening my excessive alcohol drinking and lack of sleep from the previous night triggered hypomania.

On our wedding night at a local bed-and-breakfast, I was exhausted, but I remained awake, my thoughts racing. I had no idea what was going on with my brain. The next day while speaking with my mother on the phone, she asked if Pat had us sign the marriage certificate. When I told her we hadn't signed it yet, I didn't expect her to become so upset over Pat's ineptitude. She was irrational and hysterical. I responded to her overreaction by yelling so loudly that my throat bled and the dogs pressed against my legs in alarm. Crying, I hung up the phone. Craig was in another room when he heard the commotion. As he helped me calm down, he didn't voice his concern about my worrisome outburst. I was so drained, I didn't know if I'd be able to go on our honeymoon to the Sierras.

My behavior was due to hypomania. While hypomania is often associated with euphoria, it can include agitation. Agitation may manifest as excessive talking or unintentional and purposeless motions, i.e. wringing of the hands or pacing. Other symptoms include hostility, uncooperativeness, and disruptive behavior. I slept well the next two nights, and the hypomania subsided. But I didn't breathe a word about the racing thoughts I had during our wedding night. It was an unnerving memory, and I wanted to forget it had ever happened.

After my marriage certificate meltdown, my brain settled down over the next year. I felt ready to take on a job and I scanned the newspaper's classified section. My shoulder muscles ached with exasperation over the slim pickings. The word had gotten out through the internet about Santa Cruz's breathtaking beauty and the dynamic community, and local employment opportunities had become scarce. When I read an advertisement for an administrative assistant at a California State Parks-affiliated non-profit, my skills matched the job's requirements. Ever since I moved to Santa Cruz, I loved visiting the Santa Cruz County state parks. The job would not be my dream career, but work would anchor me. When I was asked to interview at Friends of Santa Cruz State Parks, I was going to do my best to get the job.

At my interview, I dressed up in one of my Downtown Association suits and looked professional, but I was a nervous wreck. My stomach was so queasy, I worried I'd have to sprint for the restroom. I had no reason to be anxious. I had a great education, diverse administrative work experience, and glowing referrals. Nevertheless, the interview panel intimidated me. The Executive Director and three board members took turns inquiring about my work experience and my reasons for wanting the position. My voice shook as I answered the questions. When I walked out the door, I felt ashamed for botching the interview.

Two days later, I received a voicemail from the Friends of Santa Cruz State Parks' coordinator Melissa. I anticipated a rejection, but Melissa's voice sounded cheerful. She told me I had been selected for the position. I thought she had mixed me up with another candidate! Melissa mentored me and became a friend. Working with her reminded me of my positive experience with Sharon at Silicon Events. While my pay was low given my responsibilities, I received health benefits, and I set up my first 401(k) retirement savings plan. My other coworkers and the Board of Directors were passionate about the local state parks and treated their roles with pride. I envied them for having found their calling.

Will I ever figure out what I want to do? I wondered.

Two years passed by uneventfully. During my time at the non-profit, I had another, secret job: hiding my depressed mood from the workplace. I assumed my depression lingered because I hadn't found my identity or my dream job. I thought being married would melt away my dejection, but our marriage couldn't fix an unremitting mood disorder. Soon after I turned thirty, I received pregnancy announcements from several women I knew. I too wanted to be a mother, and Craig wanted to be a father, but we hadn't discussed a specific timeline for our plans.

Spring arrived, and my depression lightened up with the warm weather. One evening after Craig returned home from work, I handed him a glass of Merlot wine. I asked him to sit down. I never greeted him with drinks, and I couldn't hide my ear-to-ear grin, so it only took him a second to figure out I was pregnant. Once his initial shock wore off, he joined me in my excitement and gave me a long, tight hug.

As with most other pregnant mothers, I worried about the health of our baby and how my labor would turn out, especially since I was on the older side at age thirty-four. For a worrywart like myself, pregnancy offers all kinds of things to fret and obsess over. To reduce my fears of the unknown, I researched a variety of birth topics and came across the subject of doulas. Doulas are trained professionals who assist women during and after childbirth. They are often hired when a couple has no immediate family available to help them after their child is born. I was excited to find a non-profit organization that offered doula services at a significant discount. If we were accepted into their program, I'd be assigned a senior doula and a trainee. My application was approved, and we were paired with an experienced doula named Liz and her trainee Kristina.

We arranged for Liz and Kristina to meet with us before my due date so we'd get acquainted. My ultrasound showed we were having a girl whom we named Avonlea, which means river meadow in Old English. I found the name in L.M. Montgomery's classic *Anne of Green Gables*, one of my most treasured books. We were on our way to having our baby join us, and I was more excited, scared, and hopeful than I had ever been before.

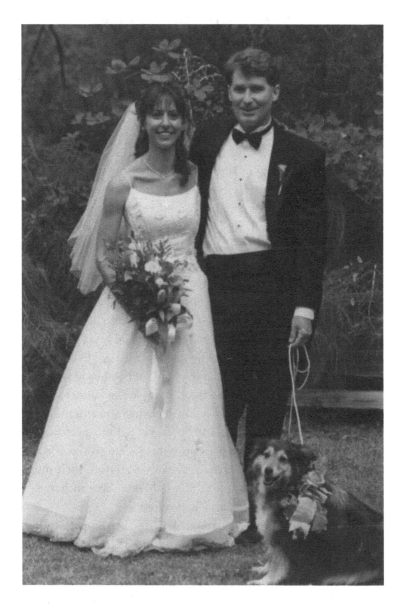

Our wedding at Quail Hollow Ranch, Felton, California, October 2001

CHAPTER THIRTEEN

A Hint of What's to Come

On a rainy evening in January 2005, I was splayed out on the couch watching television—all 180 pounds of me. I felt a series of uncomfortable cramps. When I realized they were labor contractions, I panicked. Sheets of rain began falling, and the wind whipped the trees back and forth. I called Liz. She thought it was too early to go to the hospital, yet unwise for us to stay at our isolated cabin. She suggested we gather at her son Peter's house located a few blocks from the hospital. Liz's idea didn't sound appealing, but I knew it would be foolish to ignore her advice.

We arrived at Peter's house at midnight, and I was shown to a bedroom where Liz suggested I lie down. As I stood by the bed, I felt a warm popping sensation in my belly. My amniotic sac broke and gushed clear fluid onto the floor. That gave us cause to get to the Sutter Maternity Hospital because during a prenatal exam I had tested positive for group B strep. It was Sutter's protocol for a patient with group B strep to go immediately to the hospital once the amniotic sac had broken. When we arrived, I felt much better being in a modern, clean hospital room, and in between contractions I breathed a deep sigh of relief!

I had planned to labor without the aid of pain medication. Within a few minutes of meeting Liz and Kristina for the first time, Liz voiced her dogmatic opposition to using epidurals for childbirth pain. She had a wealth of experience—she had attended two hundred and sixty-two births. Liz's staunch opinion influenced me, and I adopted her philosophy. But after my labor had begun, I was in excruciating pain throughout the night. Kristina volunteered to walk with me through the hallways to move along my labor. I barely knew Kristina and I felt uncomfortable clutching her arm, especially when I doubled over in pain. What Liz, Kristina, Craig, and I didn't know was my staying up all night had triggered hypomania.

In the morning I began the homestretch to birth. I couldn't believe how much the contractions hurt.

"Please, PLEASE get me some pain relief," I wailed.

"It's too late to get an epidural," Liz said tersely. I wasn't thrilled with her response and came close to firing her as my doula. Our spunky nurse Mary told me I could have intravenous Fentanyl. Liz didn't say a word. She knew I might bite off her head if she did.

"Fentanyl will take the edge off the pain," Mary reassured me. I waited for the Fentanyl to arrive with bated breath!

Soon after I became pregnant with Avonlea, Craig and I decided on using a team of reputable certified nurse-midwives at Sutter Maternity Hospital. Our decision caused concern among our family members who preferred medical doctors. However, I learned that, unlike most obstetricians, certified nurse-midwives are registered nurses who have close relationships with their patients. If complications arise during pregnancy or labor, they work in tandem with obstetricians. Sutter Maternity Hospital was an ideal place to have a baby. The building was only a few years old, and our airy room on the second floor had a large window that faced eucalyptus tree-covered hills. My health insurance covered all costs except for a three-hundred-dollar co-payment. There was a daybed for Craig and a rocking chair, plus a bathroom and tub.

Craig didn't want to be at what he called the "business end" during childbirth. He was certain he could never cut an umbilical cord. I didn't mind his decision. But when the moment of Avonlea's birth drew near, and I was "open for business," Craig saw the amazed expressions of our midwife, nurse, and doulas, and he changed his mind. I was thrilled he wanted to observe his daughter the moment she was born. Craig watched Avonlea emerge to give her first bellowing cry.

As Avonlea was gently placed on my chest, Nurse Mary asked Craig, "Aren't you going to cut the cord?"

"Uh, I hadn't planned on it," he said as I kissed Avonlea's soft cheek.

When I was given Avonlea to hold, she was covered with vernix, a slippery substance. Vernix serves the purpose of moisturizing and protecting the skin and helps babies to move through the birth canal. After Craig informed Mary he wasn't cutting the cord, she made fun of his queasiness.

"Buk buk buk brr-awk!" Mary clucked like a chicken.

The excitement wasn't over yet.

I was astonished when Mary handed a pair of scissors to *me* to cut the cord, although my shaky arms held a slippery baby. Craig's eyes widened in disbelief, and in a split second he grabbed the scissors and cut the cord.

I was delirious with joy over Avonlea's birth. I had a huge smile, but I looked creepy. My eyes' capillaries had burst during labor because I held my breath during each push, and as a result, the whites of my eyes were bright red. Although my hypomania had begun, it was undetected by all. The happiness I felt as I held my baby girl was authentic. I was grateful to feel connected to Avonlea from the start, and I had no tinges of postpartum depression, although hours earlier, Nurse Mary had read my medical history chart that mentioned my clinical depression. Before we were discharged, she took Craig aside. She told him to make sure I got enough sleep and rest to stave off postpartum depression.

In 2005, many new fathers had no awareness of perinatal mood and anxiety disorders, and Craig was one of them. Nurse Mary's advice got his attention, and Craig observed my behavior at home. After Avonlea was born, Craig noticed I had a lot of energy. I breastfed Avonlea at all hours of the day and night. Craig didn't regard my behavior as extreme enough for psychiatric attention, but he became frustrated. My weary, exasperated husband was burning the candle at both ends. He did the majority of the nighttime diaper changes, and his geological engineering job was stressful. His aggravation with my hyperactivity turned into anger.

When Craig had reached his limit, he yelled, "Dyane, that's it—if you don't rest like the nurse said, I'm buying a case of formula and you're going to sleep during the night!"

I knew my husband wasn't trying to control me—he wanted to take care of our family. He was not the yelling type. I tried to sleep, but my hypomania was still active, and it was responsible for my making a scene in public when Avonlea was two weeks old.

The first time a mother goes on an outing without her newborn is usually challenging. My first baby-free excursion was not only difficult, but I conducted myself in a ridiculous, hypomanic-fueled manner. Before I knew Avonlea's due date, I bought two concert tickets for my musical heroes, the New Zealand-born brothers Neil and Tim Finn. The show was on Valentine's Day at the historic Palace of Fine Arts Theatre in San Francisco. After Avonlea was born, I assumed I'd give the tickets away and stay home, but Craig knew how much seeing the duo would mean to me. He encouraged me to go to the show with my friend Yvette, and offered to care for Avonlea. I wanted to see the Finn Brothers perform so badly, but I could barely stand the thought of leaving my baby for ten minutes, let alone four hours. I pumped enough milk so Craig could feed Avonlea in my absence.

On Valentine's Day, a heavy rain began falling in the late afternoon. Driving in the rain always made me nervous, and I was tempted to cancel my plans. As Avonlea napped, Craig looked at my anxious face and gave me a hug.

"Dyane, you'll be fine," he said. "Once you're at the concert, you won't regret it. The hardest part is walking out the door!"

As a longtime fan, I wanted to give the Finn Brothers tokens of appreciation. They were avid cold water surfers, and I came up with the perfect gift: two copies of *Mavericks* by Matt Warshaw. The coffee-table book features jaw-dropping pictures of the enormous surf break in Half Moon Bay, California. I daydreamed about handing the books to the musicians and seeing their faces light up.

At the Palace of Fine Arts, the performance was fantastic even though Neil sounded like a frog. He apologized to the audience for his croaky singing and explained he had a cold. After the show, I joined the other fans at the stage exit and we stood in the pouring rain. Images of baby Avonlea's adorable face flooded my mind. I chomped at the bit to deliver the gifts quickly so we could take off. Yvette was tired, and I assured her as soon as I completed my mission, we'd be out of there.

Neil emerged from the exit and walked toward us looking worn out. Despite being near my musical hero, the last thing I wanted to do was to catch his germs and pass them on to my newborn! Neil was known for being exceptionally kind to his fans. While I appreciated his graciousness, when he stood before me, I leaned away from him as I handed him the book. I didn't listen to a thing he said.

Tim Finn wasn't like his genial younger brother. He strode past us, and he didn't make eye contact with anyone. I was annoyed with his demeanor, but I was unaware Tim suffered from chronic panic attacks. As I watched him walk towards the tour van, I thought, *I've left my baby at home, I've come all this way, and I'm giving this gift to Tim Finn now, dammit!*

I made a beeline for Tim. No security guard attempted to stop me. Mouth agape, Yvette watched the spectacle along with the rest of the crowd, but she didn't think any harm would come to me.

In the way only a hypomanic mother could do, I yelled at the top of my lungs, "GIFT FOR TIM FINN! GIFT FOR TIM FINN!"

I expected Tim would stop, but he didn't. I reached him the moment before he stepped into the van and I thrust the *Mavericks* book toward him. He took the gift and stared at me with ice-blue eyes. At that point, I knew Tim's parting words wouldn't be what I had imagined in my Day-Glo fantasies.

"You're too much. You're too much," he said disparagingly in a crisp New Zealand accent.

He recognized a hypomanic fan when he saw one.

I returned home disgraced, but my humiliation vanished the moment I held my baby. I swore I'd never leave her for longer than ten minutes again! At least my intense emotions and physical exertion had one significant benefit: I got much more sleep over the next few nights. My hypomania wound itself down, and the beast of bipolar disorder wouldn't emerge until two and a half years later when Marilla was born.

CHAPTER FOURTEEN

The Depths of Despair

"You're not eating anything," said Marilla sharply, eying her as if it were a serious shortcoming. Anne sighed.

"I can't. I'm in the depths of despair. Can you eat when you are in the depths of despair?"

"I've never been in the depths of despair, so I can't say," responded Marilla.

"Weren't you? Well, did you ever try to IMAGINE you were in the depths of despair?"

"No, I didn't."

"Then I don't think you can understand what it's like. It's a very uncomfortable feeling indeed."

L.M. Montgomery, *Anne of Green Gables*

When I admitted myself to the Behavioral Health Unit six weeks after Marilla's birth, my mania was tempered by two powerful medications. I resumed taking the atypical antipsychotic olanzapine twice a day to treat my bipolar disorder, postpartum onset. I was prescribed the non-benzodiazepine zolpidem tartrate to promote sleep.

Besides Dr. King, I met with a psychiatrist named Dr. Barrington. The physician repulsed me because of his arrogance and lack of compassion. Dr. Barrington strutted around the unit in an expensive Armani charcoal suit and tie. His dark hair was stylishly cut, and when he walked by me, the smell of his vetiver aftershave lingered in the air. As much as Dr. Barrington annoyed me, I couldn't ignore his impressive Ivy League education, and I paid attention to his medical opinion because my two girls depended on me to get better.

Dr. Barrington discussed the risks of breastfeeding while taking my medications, and he recommended I stop breastfeeding to stabilize the mania. I knew it was essential to cease tandem breastfeeding Marilla and Avonlea, but it was a heartbreaking decision. Dr. Barrington warned me about the importance of remaining on the medications post-discharge.

"Mrs. Harwood, I want to be very clear that if you stop taking these medications, it would be like taking down a wall holding back a dam, and I'd expect you'd return to a more manic state within twenty-four hours," he said in a sobering tone.

"I *must* get better—I won't stop taking them," I agreed, willing to do anything so I could return to my family.

After four monotonous days at the unit, Craig and the girls arrived to take me home. As soon as we emerged into the daylight and fresh air, I took a deep breath. To be with my baby, my toddler, and my husband, and sleep in my soft bed was nothing short of miraculous.

My discharge report stated I had an "excellent expected outcome with follow-up," and I expected it would be the only psychiatric hospitalization I'd ever have. However, it was only the beginning of my psychiatric revolving door syndrome, a medical term that describes patients who endure a cyclical pattern of short-term readmissions to psychiatric units.

Upon my return home, my mania faded like a dissolving sunset. I was grateful to hold my girls and be with my husband, but my fierce love for my family didn't stop a horrendous depression from overtaking me. The combination of the antipsychotic and sleep medication I took caused massive fatigue. Each day my despair grew worse.

Soon after my discharge, I received a phone call from my mother.

"Honey, let me come up and be with you and the girls," she said in her most loving, soothing voice.

"Yes, that would be good," I mumbled. I knew I sounded terrible, but I was beyond the point of caring about how I presented myself.

Although Mom and I inevitably fought when we were together, I hoped she'd see the severity of my depression and make it a priority to comfort me. Craig and I weren't sure where she'd stay. Our house didn't have a guest room, and my mother was used to high-end hotels. Couch surfing was *not* an option! I remembered passing a "Felton Inn" sign on the highway near my home. When I looked at the Felton Inn's website, I read a testimonial from Lindsay Wagner, the actress known for her role in the television show *The Bionic Woman*. It seemed likely if Felton Inn had impressed a celebrity, it would be nice enough for Mom. The owner Holly was friendly on the phone, and she and Mom enjoyed spending time together. During their chats, my mother voiced her fears to Holly about my depression.

Every time the girls and I visited my mom at the Felton Inn, I was embarrassed to interact with vivacious Holly, who was in her early sixties but looked ten years younger. Despite her warmth, I suspected she judged me for having depression. When we met for tea and scones in her parlor, Holly rhapsodized about the healing powers of hiking in the redwoods.

"*Ja*, I hike for hours in the forest every day!" Holly crowed in her Dutch accent with the enthusiasm one has for a hot fudge sundae. "Hiking *always* makes me feel better!"

I cringed. I couldn't imagine hiking nor could I imagine anything lifting my oppressive, hopeless mood.

It's incredibly painful for a mother to have a mentally ill child. I had ceased to be the lively daughter my mother had known for more than three decades. My bipolar diagnosis couldn't help but create profound worry and disappointment for her. Mom saw I couldn't relate to anyone, even my children and husband. She was devastated she couldn't alleviate even a small amount of my misery.

Exhausted from both my depression and medication side effects, I moved sluggishly. My new reality was a complete nightmare, and I had no idea what to do about it. What gave me the tiniest glimmer of hope was my upcoming appointment with my new psychiatrist Dr. Arana. Our latest health insurance plan didn't cover Dr. Gordon's services, and few psychiatrists in the county accepted new patients, but Dr. Arana was willing to meet with me.

Upon our first meeting, I liked the homely doctor's sense of humor and his self-deprecating manner. He reminded me of the actor Vincent Schiavelli who was known for playing the droopy-eyed psychiatric patient Fredrickson in *One Flew Over the Cuckoo's Nest*. When I left his office, my glimmer of hope had grown. But during our subsequent sessions, I was dismayed when Dr. Arana complained at length about his problems. My depression made me too meek to question his behavior. I merely sat and listened as sympathetically as I could. I wasn't speaking much given my dejection. Sometimes I thought I should be the one billing him for psychotherapy rather than the other way around.

Dr. Arana prescribed medication after medication for my depression, but nothing worked. Each time I tried a new medication, I prayed the pills would miraculously restore me to my old self. After each fruitless trial, I became more despondent. Dr. Arana and I had the same conversation following every medication's failure:

"Dr. Arana, I took the lamotrigine exactly the way I was supposed to, but I felt nothing," I said.

Dr. Arana sighed. He dug around in his messy desk drawer and handed me a packet.

"Why don't you try this sample of fluoxetine and olanzapine?"

Dr. Arana's exasperated sighs and facial expressions made it crystal clear he was frustrated to have a medication-resistant patient on his hands. His discouraging attitude only added to my hopelessness. While I knew he had good intentions, I should have found another psychiatrist after Dr. Arana's second round of sighs.

When Marilla was three months old, Dr. Arana prescribed a tricyclic antidepressant called amitriptyline. Ever since I left the Behavioral Health Unit, I took olanzapine, but it wasn't affecting my intractable depression. I hoped amitriptyline would elevate my mood. Dr. Arana never mentioned an antidepressant could send me into mania, a potentially life-threatening side effect for those with bipolar disorder. When I took amitriptyline, it did not trigger mania, but after I swallowed the harmless-looking tablet, I'd come close to losing my life.

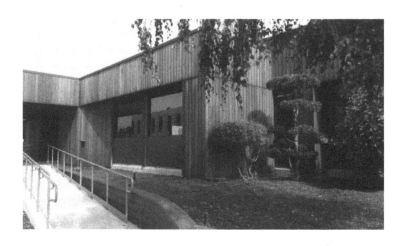

The Behavioral Health Unit had an attractive exterior, but inside it was an
austere, bleak environment.

CHAPTER FIFTEEN

One Pill Can Kill

Several hours after I had ingested amitriptyline, I felt strange. I had the strongest compulsion to kill myself that I had ever experienced in my life. I looked down at my plush green bathrobe's extra-long, thick belt and envisioned looping it around my neck and fastening the other end to our second story deck railing. Minutes passed by while I rapidly lost touch with my sense of self. My children sprawled out on the living room floor watching *The Wiggles* on television as I paced back and forth behind them. Thankfully, they were in a happy world that was the opposite of mine. As I watched my daughters enjoy the wacky Australian pop singers, my connection to reality dwindled. Two thoughts, one rational and one deadly, battled against one another in my mind:

You don't want to leave your girls—you can't do it!

I must hang myself.

Before I took amitriptyline, I had never considered taking my life by asphyxiation. I couldn't comprehend why anyone would want to do such a barbaric act when there were less excruciating methods of self-annihilation. It seemed logical that amitriptyline had triggered my suicidal ideation. Amitriptyline has been prescribed for decades, and there has been a long-standing concern among psychiatrists that as an antidepressant, it has a suicide risk. There is no doubt about it: psychiatric medication can be one's salvation *or* poison. Ideally, a person who is undergoing treatment for a mood disorder needs to be monitored once *any* pill enters the bloodstream, either by loved ones or in a hospital, over a period of days. The truth of the matter is many people have to go it alone when trying new medications.

The day my medicine became my poison, Craig was working at home. If he hadn't been nearby, I might have gone beyond the edge of reason and left my family forever. As I stood near the girls, petrified, Craig walked into the room. He took one look at my distraught face, grabbed my hand, and pulled me into the kitchen.

"Dyane, what's going on?" he asked softly so Avonlea and Marilla wouldn't become alarmed. I couldn't meet his eyes.

"Something's wrong! Something's wrong with me—I need to get to the hospital," I stuttered. I was still lucid enough to know the girls could hear me, so I refrained from mentioning my suicide plan.

Craig gathered every bit of strength he had to make another drive to a psychiatric unit. Once again, bipolar disorder would be responsible for dividing a family. Once again I'd go to a sterile, soulless unit where I'd feel devoid of hope and terrified. We had no savings and our health insurance only covered some psychiatric care. While I knew we'd receive another astronomical bill for my hospitalization, there would be nothing we could do but set up a payment plan and worry about finances later.

While Craig got the girls ready to pile into our Subaru Outback, he asked me to call hospitals in our county to see if a bed was available. Because he still didn't know the specifics of my agonizing thoughts, he thought I'd be able to use the phone and speak coherently to a stranger. Miraculously, I had the presence of mind to call the Behavioral Health Unit, but it was full, so I contacted a Monterey hospital where I was connected to a sympathetic nurse. After I told her I was feeling suicidal and had a baby and toddler, she said they had one bed left and she promised she'd hold it for me. She spoke briefly with Craig to make sure the kids were safe, and we headed south for the hospital.

When I said a quick goodbye to Craig and our girls at the emergency room, it was one of the worst moments of my life.

I couldn't look at Avonlea and Marilla's faces for longer than a moment for fear of sobbing hysterically. I was handed off to a tall attendant named Malosi who led me to the Marine Parade, the hospital's absurd euphemism for its psychiatric unit. We stopped by a water fountain and Malosi offered me a tranquilizer. Although he could pass for a linebacker, Malosi had a gentle manner and said warmly, "It'll help with anxiety." I nodded yes, and he handed me a tiny paper cup containing the benzodiazepine lorazepam. It was the first benzodiazepine I had ever taken and was known for being a fast-acting medication. I gulped the pill down, praying it would lessen my intense fear.

When Malosi and I reached the Marine Parade, we paused in front of the unit's locked door. As he pressed the entrance button to speak with a nurse, I shook with a degree of panic lorazepam couldn't quell. A loud buzz sounded that allowed us to enter, and we walked into the community room, a bleak area filled with beige utilitarian tables. White-gowned patients were eating dinner, but I had no appetite and declined the meal. I didn't look at anyone as I passed through the community room. Malosi and I reached the unit's main corridor and walked until he stopped at the doorway of a small room with a single bed.

"Thank you, Malosi," I said weakly.

"You'll feel better soon," he replied and flashed me a smile. Malosi turned around and walked away. Bereft of hope, I was on my own.

The lorazepam had made me woozy, and I was relieved I didn't need to share my space. Even in my detached state, I knew a single room was a luxury at any psychiatric unit. The next day I slowly wandered around the Marine Parade in a daze. There wasn't much to explore—there were the patients' bedrooms, the community room, a doctor's office, and a group therapy room. As with the Behavioral Health Unit staff, Monterey's personnel offered occupational therapy (O.T.) for making crafts. I was familiar with O.T. long before my hospitalizations took place. Once after my father had been discharged from the Neuropsychiatric Institute, he brought home a vase he made in O.T. I could tell his depression had lifted because he jokingly referred to his craft as the "ten-thousand-dollar vase," the cost of his brief time at the hospital.

On my first full day at the Marine Parade, I sat at a table in front of a basket filled with colored pencil stubs and dog-eared coloring books. Although other patients sat nearby, I made no attempt to talk with them. In the past when I was healthy, I could easily strike up conversations with almost anyone. I wanted to make people around me feel welcome. After what happened with amitriptyline, I was demoralized and no longer felt human. All I wanted to do was disappear.

I noticed the other patients had enough focus and drive to create leather belts. I couldn't picture myself making a bed, let alone a complex-looking belt. I was so depressed I could barely pick up a pencil, but I forced myself to take one from the basket to color a mermaid picture. After I walked away from my first O.T. session, I felt ashamed and thought, *I've gone from being a college graduate, an employee, a wife, and a mom to someone I don't recognize.*

Over the next few days as the amitriptyline was flushed out of my system, I was given new medication. My suicidal ideation was no longer acute, but I was still deeply depressed. Our large chunks of free time did nothing to hasten our recovery. There were barely any books or magazines to read. In my suicidal state, I hadn't thought to pack any reading material. The staff didn't escort patients for outdoor walks, which deprived us of the fresh air and sunlight that could have helped improve our moods.

Ironically, the hospital had beautiful grounds perfect for outings, and it overlooked one of the world's most magnificent coastlines, but patients were kept inside.

I had read about psychiatric units that offered healing modalities such as animal therapy, music, and much more, but the Marine Parade was a bare-bones program. When I was there, patients had no internet access or cellular phone use, so I was cut off from emails, texts, and online sources of encouragement such as virtual support groups and blogs. The unit's thick windows were glazed with security glass, and the stale air and fluorescent lighting made it a drab place to be.

I met with Dr. Adelstein, the Marine Parade's chief psychiatrist. Dr. Adelstein was a soft-spoken, modest man who resembled the dark-haired actor Robert Downey Jr. My week at the Marine Parade helped me get stable enough to return home. I continued suffering from bipolar depression, but my acute suicidal ideation was gone. After I had gone to the hideously dark place of suicidal ideation, I developed a deep empathy for those who feel suicidal and who die by suicide. I wanted to believe I had fulfilled my lifetime's quota of suffering and hoped I'd never visit the hell of suicidal ideation again. But I couldn't predict and prevent the tragic losses headed my way. Many resilient people are wired so they don't fall apart when beset by grief. I knew I wasn't one of them. It would be only a matter of time when I'd face great loss, and when that time came, I'd do something I never thought I would do in order to survive.

CHAPTER SIXTEEN

Making Medication My Enemy

After my discharge from the Marine Parade unit, my life was in shambles. The lack of structure to my days did nothing to improve my depression. I felt guilty I wasn't able to hold down a job and contribute to our household, but Craig never made me feel bad about my unemployment. I was fortunate to have a loving husband supporting our family. Working would have been impossible—I had no motivation to climb out of my mental morass.

Over the next ten months, I remained despondent. Despite trying gabapentin, divalproex sodium, paroxetine, fluoxetine, quetiapine, duloxetine, amitriptyline, lamotrigine, risperidone, and other medications, my depression didn't budge. My desperation drove me to research alternative modalities that could lift bipolar depression.

I asked Dr. Arana, "Have you seen the holistic approach work for anyone?" He gave me a skeptical look.

"Dyane, alternative treatments have *never* helped my patients," Dr. Arana said. It was dispiriting to hear his response, and I didn't bring up the topic with him again.

However, that session was a significant turning point. I stopped being passive and read about alternative treatment options on the internet. At first, I could barely concentrate, but my focus improved little by little. I read while my girls attended preschool when the house was quiet. I was interested in any simple regimen, such as light therapy. Light therapy was ideal since all it involved was

sitting in front of a therapeutic light. I already owned a SunBox®
light I had purchased before Avonlea's birth. I read psychiatrist Dr.
Norman Rosenthal groundbreaking bestseller *Winter Blues* about
using light therapy for Seasonal Affective Disorder and other mood
disorders. I sat in front of my light each morning and followed
Dr. Rosenthal's guidelines for safe, effective use of the SunBox.
For some people with bipolar disorder, light therapy can cause
hypomania or mania. It's important to be aware of the risk, find
out the latest medical recommendations, and discuss light therapy
with your doctor. Fortunately, I never experienced hypomania or
mania when using my light.

Sitting in front of my SunBox was not only painless and
effortless; it gave me a sense of accomplishment. While light
therapy alone would not get my mood where it needed to be, it
was a good place to begin. Based on everything I'd learned from
being a certified personal trainer, exercise had to be part of the
equation. My energy level was low, and I needed something easy
to do, so I chose walking. We lived near Highlands Park, an area
with a short nature trail loop. Twenty minutes a day, I walked the
Highlands loop as if I were in a trance. I was a far cry from the
Banana Slug Fitness trainer I had been a decade earlier. Although
my depression made me pessimistic, when I walked I noticed
the beauty of the trees, flowers, and burbling San Lorenzo River
rushing alongside the trail. The air was brisk and smelled good,
and I soaked up the natural daylight.

I continued reading articles and anecdotes about supplements
that allegedly helped lift bipolar depression. A small-scale pilot
study found that high doses of fish oil with omega-3 fatty acids
significantly improved bipolar depression symptoms. I stared at
images of golden-colored fish oil capsules on my computer screen
until my eyes were blurry from fatigue. Avonlea and Marilla
played with their toys on the living room floor as I scanned page

after page of omega-3 testimonials. I took a break to gaze out the window and reflect upon what I had read.

Maybe there's a chance for me if I use this supplement. I'm not taking a risk like I did with amitriptyline—no one has died from fish oil. The worst side effect is an upset stomach. God knows I could handle that!

I requested a library copy of Harvard psychiatrist Dr. Andrew Stoll's bestselling book *The Omega-3 Connection: The Groundbreaking Anti-Depression Diet and Brain Program*. After I had read it, I was certain I needed to try fish oils. I was interested in using Nordic Naturals, a leading fish oil manufacturer and a local company. However, before I could buy my first bottle, I had to overcome a major hurdle. Quality fish oil supplements were expensive, especially the Nordic Naturals potent liquid product I wanted. I was broke, and there was only one person I could think of who I could ask for financial help: my mother. Pacing back and forth in the kitchen, I picked up the phone and forced myself to dial my parents' number.

"Hi, Mom. It's me," I said timidly.

"Are you okay? Are the girls okay?" she asked, her voice filled with concern.

"Yes, yes, everyone is fine, Mom. I'm calling because I want to buy liquid fish oil, but it's expensive. It's safe, and it could help me feel better." I could hear my mother sigh as I spoke, her television blaring the QVC shopping channel in the background.

"Are you *sure* it's safe with the medication you're taking?" she asked.

"Yes! A Harvard psychiatrist recommends fish oil for bipolar disorder, Mom," I said. Dr. Stoll's position and reputation would go a long way in calming her anxiety about the supplements.

"Dyane, you know my finances are tight," she said.

I gulped. I *hated* asking her for money, but I had to swallow my pride if I wanted to start swallowing fish oil!

"Go ahead and order the fish oil. I'll reimburse you," she said hurriedly. "I have someone on the other line, I think it's my doctor, so I'll talk to you later, honey." Before I could say "Thank you!" I heard a dial tone. As uncomfortable as it was to ask for my mother's help, I was grateful to receive her financial support. Many people don't have a parent who's willing to foot the bill for supplements.

Worrying about interactions between my medication and fish oil wouldn't be a concern because I had stopped taking my medication. I kept my decision secret because if Dr. Arana found out, he could claim I was a danger to myself and others, and hospitalize me against my will. I didn't cease taking my medication cold turkey because that was a dangerous risk. Instead, I spoke with Dr. Arana about tapering the aripiprazole I had been prescribed and I told him I'd resume taking lithium, but I didn't intend to carry that out. After seven weeks of tapering off aripiprazole, my depression diminished. Two weeks later, I woke up and realized, to my amazement, my depression had disappeared. I went to wake up Avonlea and Marilla, who were used to my morose morning expression. Upon seeing my smile, they gave me big hugs. Craig was at a remote job site that didn't have cell phone reception, but I'd speak with him when got home.

I wanted to share my news with someone who would be thrilled for me, and my friend Sharon came to mind.

"Dyane, I'm so happy for you—the old you is back!" she said. We made plans to get together for a walk.

My mother also noticed the shift in my mood. "You seem like you're doing much better," she said, relief permeating her voice. When Craig came home, I had a change of heart about telling him about my depression's disappearance. I had a feeling he'd figure out I had ceased taking meds, he'd get angry, and he'd oppose my decision. We only spoke for a few minutes before he holed up in his office to work on reports. The rest of the evening, I dialed down my ebullience.

I met with Dr. Arana that week, and asked him, "Do you think I'm manic?"

"I don't know," he said.

Dr. Arana's uncertainty perplexed me. I also questioned his competency. He had been put on probation by the medical board for overprescribing to patients. I grew defensive as I walked out of his office and rationalized, *He should know if I'm manic! But this goes to show that psychiatrists don't know everything. I should be able to go off meds without feeling like I need his approval.*

After trying more than twenty psychiatric drugs, I was completely burned out. The atypical antipsychotic medication I most recently took, aripiprazole, turned me into a lethargic, hopeless woman. After scrutinizing holistic healing success stories, I was compelled to pursue alternative healing. I placed my first order and hoped the fish oil would prevent the return of my depression.

After Federal Express delivered my fish oil, I eagerly opened the box. I measured my first dose of fish oil and tried my best not to spill an expensive drop. The thick, opaque liquid tasted fishy, which made sense. The formulation contained lemon, but it didn't mask the fishy flavor. As I placed my bottles of "liquid gold" into the refrigerator, Craig wandered into the kitchen.

"What's that?" he asked as he stared at my twisted-up mouth.

"Remember the book I read about fish oils helping bipolar depression?" I said offhandedly. "Mom treated me to fish oil—it's safe for me to take it."

Craig didn't ask me if I was taking my medication. He trusted me. I hated deceiving him, but I felt I had no other option—the quality of my life was at stake. That night we joined Avonlea and Marilla in the living room. Our girls danced wildly with one another to the goofy children's television show *Yo Gabba Gabba!*

As I looked at my daughters' joyful faces, I prayed my brain would stop making my life hell so I could be a better mother.

Besides subsidizing the fish oil, my mom sent me a small check so I could treat myself to a new shirt or dress. Before my diagnosis, I would have loved to buy a cute outfit. Now, I wanted something more practical. I wanted pills, but not the pharmacological kind. I had read articles about an intriguing-sounding herbal supplement called holy basil. Holy basil (tulsi) has been used in India for centuries. Ayurvedic masters recommend the herb for encouraging a healthy mood. Modern-day users of holy basil write about its calming, balancing effects. Holy basil sounded like an ideal supplement and there didn't seem to be a catch. The only adverse side effect I read about was the herb's anti-fertility effect, which wasn't a concern as our family was complete. I used Mom's gift money at the health food store, where I quizzed the staff on which holy basil brand was the best. I added a bottle of Organic India® capsules to my holistic arsenal.

I believed with all my might my healthy lifestyle would prevent the onslaught of depression. I was convinced I was in control of my body, but I was not. I knew how to strengthen a muscle, but I didn't know how to keep my mood from soaring too high or plummeting too low. As much as I wanted my brain synapses to settle, it was too late for that now.

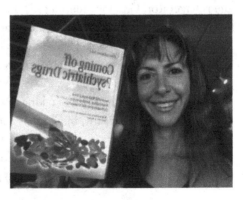

I used a psychiatric medication-tapering book to guide me, but despite my best efforts, I became hypomanic and relapsed.

CHAPTER SEVENTEEN

Found Out

My favorite month of October had arrived, and I continued keeping my med-free decision a secret from Craig. He still hadn't asked me why I seemed so much happier. Later, he would tell me he suspected something was amiss, but his stressful workload distracted him. He was exhausted whenever we crossed paths, which wasn't often. We had become the proverbial ships passing in the night. I didn't press for more time together because when I looked at his weary face, I felt guilty for lying to him. I grew paranoid he'd find out about my deception. When the girls were playing Sequence, one of their favorite board games, I took Craig aside. He beat me to the punch.

"You're off your medication, aren't you?" he said, looking exasperated and angry.

"Just hear me out—please? Imagine forcing someone who has diabetes to eat a bag of sugar, which makes her sick. I feel like that person. People are demanding I take meds that make me feel terrible. Does that make any sense?" I asked him.

"No, it makes absolutely no sense," he said adamantly.

I presented another angle, pleading, "It takes time for any medication to work for bipolar—at least a couple weeks for most of the meds. It has only been five weeks since I started the supplements. It's too soon to tell if all these alternative things are taking effect!"

"Sorry, Dyane. I don't buy it! You're hypomanic." Craig said.

Despite using light therapy, walking, taking fish oil and holy basil, when I stopped my medication, I induced my hypomania. I slept much less than usual. For most people with bipolar disorder, adequate sleep is the linchpin for mood stability. When my sleep dropped to three or four hours a night, a relapse was imminent.

On a mild October afternoon, I turned on Craig's iMac computer to format a support group flyer. Courtesy of hypomania's inspiration, I had decided to create a "Moms with Bipolar" support group. The iMac was connected to our printer, and I wanted to print a master copy of my flyer. Craig's email program automatically opened, and I spotted my name in the subject header of several emails exchanged between Craig and my brother. I couldn't resist opening one. The content completely undid me.

Craig wrote, "Thanks for checking in. Dyane's mental state is getting worse. I'm at a total loss as to what I can do—the only thing I can think of is to give her an ultimatum. I'll have to bring up separating unless she resumes taking her medication."

Reading Craig's email made me feel nauseous, and I hyperventilated. One of my greatest fears was my husband leaving me. To discover he was considering separation got me so upset, I couldn't sleep that night. The sleep deprivation intensified my hypomania and primed me for a manic outburst.

The following day I raced around the house preparing to host a baby playgroup. Craig had the day off from work, and I buried my fury behind a phony smile that made my face ache. At 10:00 a.m., a bevy of babies, toddlers, and moms filled up our living room. Craig took off for a hike. Even though I was anxious and exhausted, I kept up my cheery facade. After the playgroup had ended, our house was a mess. I should have asked the moms to clean up, but I didn't want to impose upon them. I was frantically straightening up the living room when Craig walked through the door.

"Dyane, this place looks like a tornado blew through it!"

In a flash, I lost my temper. I yelled at him using my raunchiest vocabulary words. Marilla was secure in her baby chair, and Avonlea was watching television. Both girls cried when they heard my enraged voice. During the past week when I was agitated around Craig, he had warned me if I acted out of control, he'd call the police to ask for a "wellness check." A visit from the police could lead to an officer placing me under a 5150 psychiatric hold to hospitalize me for mania. A 5150, a California legal code, authorizes an officer to involuntarily confine a person suspected to have a mental disorder that makes her a danger to herself or to others. If given a 5150, not only would I be hospitalized for a minimum of 72 hours, I'd be pressured by doctors to resume taking the psychotropic drugs I believed were causing my bipolar depression. True to his word, when I yelled at him, Craig picked up the phone.

Furious, I chased my husband around the house. We were in the bedroom out of the girls' sight when I ripped a hole in his T-shirt and punched him in the shoulder. It was the first time during our relationship I was violent. Hitting Craig indicated my mental stability was deteriorating, especially since I grew up terrified by domestic violence. I had sworn my children would never be in a house with such frightening madness, yet I was going against what I believed in the most.

It only took a few minutes for four police officers to appear on our doorstep. The officers separated us so they could hear our sides of the story, and Craig took the girls downstairs. I waited in the living room until the police could interview me about what happened.

"Mrs. Harwood, could you please explain why your husband's shirt is torn?" the senior officer asked me. To avoid being hospitalized, I realized I needed to deny my impetuous behavior, but when I spoke, I sabotaged my attempt to appear innocent.

"Oh, I didn't rip his shirt, Officer," I drawled. "I'm *sure* he tore it on a redwood branch during his hike."

My explanation would have been reasonable, except for one hitch: I had crossed the line from hypomania into acute mania. Instead of treating the situation seriously, I had a smirk on my face as I spoke. The officer noticed my facial expression and heard the tone of my voice and paused.

"Mrs. Harwood, we need to bring you down to the Behavioral Health Unit for an evaluation."

Dammit! I totally blew it! I thought. Nothing seemed remotely humorous anymore.

From that point on, I made sure to appear calm. Although I was manic, I was clear-headed enough to realize the more compliant I acted, the better chance I'd have a shorter hospital stay. The police advised Craig to keep our children downstairs so they wouldn't see me get handcuffed in the doorway. The restraints were the standard policy for a 5150 hold. No fewer than three squad cars were parked in front of the driveway. That day my mania didn't erase the shame I felt from being handcuffed. I wasn't a criminal; I was suffering from a mental illness!

Before we left for the hospital, I asked the officers if I could pack a book, my SunBox light, or any of my health supplements. One policeman said glibly, "You won't be needing anything there." While the hospital would not have allowed supplements or a SunBox, they would have let me bring a book. I was so drained from the intense drama, I didn't insist on bringing reading material that would have soothed me.

I was driven to the Behavioral Health Unit, and my mania took on a devil-may-care attitude. It no longer occurred to me that if I behaved recklessly, I'd be kept longer at the hospital. After I was admitted, I met with Dr. Woodworth, a female psychiatrist who had a cold, unemotional demeanor. Dr. Woodworth told me a report would be submitted to Child Protective Services about my placing my children in danger. While I knew my girls needed a safe home environment, I thought the doctor was being rude and judgmental, and I became irate.

"Do you have children?" I asked angrily.

"No," she said.

"I can see why, you iceberg!" I yelled. I grabbed my medical file from the table and threw it against the wall. Papers flew everywhere.

My punishment was solitary confinement in a padded room for four hours. When I entered the room, which looked like a scene in *One Flew Over the Cuckoo's Nest,* I couldn't believe my surreal surroundings. There was nothing to do, but there had to be *something* I could do to forget my dehumanizing surroundings.

I sang.

I sang every Crowded House song I knew. I sang half of The Beatles' song catalog. I even sang my own compositions. I heard a deep voice from the men's unit yell, "Hey, you're pretty good!"

Someone else screamed, "Shut up! My ears are bleeding!" I sang louder.

After my punishment was complete, my voice was hoarse and my throat hurt, but as I exited the room, I exclaimed, "Never again!"

CHAPTER EIGHTEEN

Bibliotherapy and Kindred Spirits

During my hospitalization, I took an antipsychotic and a mood stabilizer to extinguish my mania. After spending six lonely, tedious days at the unit, I returned home where a profound depression descended upon me, and I could barely lift a finger to do chores. At least I was able to read, and that provided me with temporary solace.

Ever since I was a little girl, books gave me a respite from my angst. I was dyed-in-the-wool bibliophile, which means "one who loves to read, admire, and collect books." When I read an article about bibliotherapy, a form of psychotherapy that uses reading to create healing, I was intrigued. I didn't have the funds to consult a professional bibliotherapist, but I figured I could tackle a simple "do-it-yourself" bibliotherapy project. I chose uplifting novels I had enjoyed long before my diagnosis. These books had the power to transport me to another time, and they comforted me. Reading didn't cure my bipolar depression by any means, but when I immersed myself in a good book, the story often took the edge off my despair for short amounts of time.

When I was depressed, I often read L.M. Montgomery's *Emily of New Moon*. Montgomery was famous for creating the character Anne Shirley, the redheaded orphan in the 1908 classic *Anne of Green Gables*. However, Montgomery's lesser-known protagonist Emily Byrd Starr is also enchanting. The *Emily* trilogy has influenced many writers such as Madeleine L'Engle (*A Wrinkle in Time*), the author who inspired me to write. In L'Engle's book *Walking on*

Water she mentioned books she had read as a child and wrote, "My favorite was *Emily of New Moon* by Lucy Maud Montgomery, who is better known for her *Anne of Green Gables* books. I read and reread and reread *Emily of New Moon*. I liked the Anne stories, but especially I loved Emily, because she, too, wanted to be a writer, a real writer; she, too, walked to the beat of a different drum; she had a touch of second sight, that gift which allows us to peek for a moment at the world beyond ordinary space and time."

I related to the moody Emily Byrd Starr more than I did to the cheerful Anne Shirley. Emily is a passionate, talented writer. When her stern Aunt Elizabeth denies her the use of paper, Emily writes on any surface she can find, such as old-fashioned letter bills destined for the trash. Emily is obsessed with writing; sometimes it consumes her, but writing sustains her overall. Montgomery had a similar preoccupation with writing throughout her literary career.

I was fascinated with Montgomery's belief in the hereafter that she incorporated throughout the *Emily* trilogy. In *Emily of New Moon,* Emily experiences "the flash," her name for a phenomenon that gives her a magical glimpse into the afterlife. In her autobiography *The Alpine Path* Montgomery revealed she had flashes of her own. She wrote, "It has always seemed to me, ever since early childhood, that, amid all the commonplaces of life, I was very near to a kingdom of ideal beauty. Between it and me hung only a thin veil. I could never draw it quite aside, but sometimes a wind fluttered it and I caught a glimpse of the enchanting realm beyond—only a glimpse—but those glimpses have always made life worthwhile."

In *Emily of New Moon,* Emily encounters a variety of beautiful, amazing, or commonplace things in daily life that trigger the flash. But sometimes Emily's flash came upon her in unpleasant settings such as when her classmates bullied her or when she was scolded for doing something naughty. Montgomery wrote,

This moment came rarely—went swiftly, leaving her breathless with the inexpressible delight of it. She could never recall it—never summon it—never pretend it; but the wonder of it stayed with her for days. It never came twice with the same thing. Tonight the dark boughs against that far-off sky had given it. It had come with a high, wild note of wind in the night, with a shadow wave over a ripe field, with a greybird lighting on her window-sill in a storm, with the singing of 'Holy, holy, holy' in church, with a glimpse of the kitchen fire when she had come home on a dark autumn night, with the spirit-like blue of ice palms on a twilit pane, with a felicitous new word when she was writing down a 'description' of something. And always when the flash came to her Emily felt that life was a wonderful, mysterious thing of persistent beauty.

I loved reading about Emily's flash, especially because I had flashes of my own as a child. I can best describe the flashes as the antithesis of depression. Flashes are ethereal and difficult to put into words, but I experienced something akin to Emily's lifting of the veil. My flashes took place while listening to beautiful music and watching sunsets, but I only had a few of them—nowhere near the number of flashes Emily enjoys throughout the *Emily* trilogy.

In September 2008, I was online and noticed the name "L.M. Montgomery" in the news headlines section. Peering closer at the screen, I saw a picture of Montgomery's middle-aged granddaughter Kate Macdonald Butler. Butler announced to the media her family had kept a secret about her grandmother, who was one of Canada's most treasured writers and renowned for *Anne of Green Gables*. The revelation of this secret had sparked a controversy in her native Canada and beyond. Butler claimed the chronically depressed Montgomery took her life by a drug overdose. Montgomery had written in her journals about suffering from bouts of chronic depression. Butler wanted to help break apart the stigma associated with mental illness and she believed sharing the truth about her famous grandmother would make a difference. Montgomery's courageous granddaughter profoundly inspired me. Butler, an articulate, powerful speaker, brought attention to the need to help people with depression and those affected by suicide, even though she knew she'd be criticized for speaking openly about her family.

Montgomery was famous for creating characters that pursued their dreams, weathered tragedies, and never gave up hope. Her books had helped me immeasurably when I was horribly depressed. After I learned of Montgomery's tragic death, I could only hope she was free of pain, in the glorious place revealed to her by the flash.

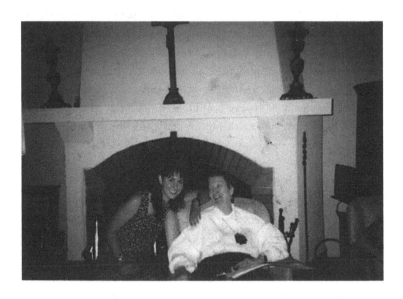

Meeting the author Madeleine L'Engle at her writer's workshop, Mount Calvary Monastery, Santa Barbara, California, late 1990s

That same year, I met another mother with bipolar disorder named Elana. She called me after spotting one of my "Moms with Bipolar" support group flyers to check if the group was still active. After I had relapsed with depression, I disbanded the group, but I hesitantly suggested we meet in a park with our kids. When Elana enthusiastically agreed to get together, I felt a slight lift in my mood, but after we had spoken, I regretted making plans with a stranger. I was depressed and anxious and I almost canceled our meeting several times. After hemming and hawing, I promised myself I would go and if I became too nervous, I'd make an early exit.

Elana and I met at the Scotts Valley Skypark where our girls could have fun in the well-equipped playground. Elana was beautiful and had a curvy figure, long auburn hair, and green eyes. She had a warm, nonjudgmental personality and a lively sense of humor. Elana was a single mother and a successful business owner. I was inspired by her confident approach to the challenges of raising a child and managing bipolar disorder. As we chatted, my girls and her daughter Sarah explored the slides and swings. When it was time to leave, Elana said it helped her to be with another mom who understood bipolar disorder. It made me feel good when she said she wanted to get together again!

In light of my heavy depression, it was significant I had shown up to meet Elana because that day I created a friendship with a kindred spirit. A kindred spirit is an old-fashioned term that describes a person who shares beliefs, attitudes, feelings, or features with another. Kindred spirits were a recurring topic in *Anne of Green Gables* and Montgomery's other books. After we spent more time together, I would discover that Elana was an extra-special kindred spirit.

As the days continued, my depression was a constant, but I was functioning. Then for no apparent reason, I became so depressed I couldn't get out of bed. Craig covered for me by taking care of our girls as best as he could, and he brought them to preschool. A trip to my psychiatrist and tweaking my medications didn't help. After wondering why I didn't return her calls, Elana unexpectedly came over to our house. I sat on the couch near her, but not too close because I was embarrassed about my grungy, unwashed body. I hadn't showered in a week, and I didn't want to do it! However, Elana was said she wasn't leaving until I took a shower. I heaved myself into the bathroom and slowly scrubbed a week's worth of sweat off my body. I'll always be grateful to my kindred spirit friend Elana. She had enough on her plate as a single mom, yet she cared enough about me to come to my house.

When depression is intractable, our friends can only do so much to help us. My anxiety and depression increased, and I became more reclusive. I couldn't handle being in public, and as bad as things were, life was about to get worse.

CHAPTER NINETEEN

Electroconvulsive Therapy to the Rescue

Electroconvulsive therapy or electroshock therapy (ECT) has been controversial since its 1934 introduction by the Hungarian neuropsychiatrist Dr. Ladislas J. Meduna. Only pure desperation would drive me to beg for electrodes to be placed on my head so that electricity would stimulate my brain.

It was January 6, 2009, fifteen months after my postpartum bipolar disorder diagnosis. I was teetering on the edge of sanity when one of my worst fears manifested.

My father died.

Dad's health had been failing for several years until he passed away, but whenever it seemed he reached his end, he'd make a miraculous recovery. But no matter how many recoveries he made, it was inevitable I'd lose him forever. Dad became frail in his seventies, and when he declined, I dreaded his death. I called him daily to cheer him up, and during our conversations, Dad shied away from talking about death-related subjects. He was terrified of dying and he was repelled by my fascination with the afterlife. I thought if he heard anecdotes of a heavenly existence, he wouldn't fear death so much. I tried swaying his opinion by telling him about two psychiatrists who believed in the hereafter: Dr. Elizabeth Kübler Ross, author of *On Death and Dying*, and Dr. Raymond Moody, author of *Life After Life*, which has sold thirteen million copies. Despite my best efforts, my tales of a great beyond fell on deaf ears, and I ceased bringing up the subject.

When I got the phone call about Dad's death, I was told he died alone in his gloomy room in a mediocre assisted living center. I became catatonic, and my depression plummeted to depths it had never reached before. After my grandmother died and I became clinically depressed, I could function. But after my father's death, my depression was much worse. Once again, I felt suicidal, and I asked Craig to take me to the Marine Parade unit. I had no plan to hurt myself, but I was devoid of hope, and I needed professional help.

Because none of the bipolar medications I tried had lifted my depression, I asked for electroconvulsive therapy (ECT). I had read articles that claimed ECT helped people with medication-resistant bipolar depression. The procedure electrically induces seizures in patients. The medical team uses anesthesia and a muscle relaxant to make ECT painless. Like many people, when I thought of ECT, I thought of the actor Jack Nicholson's character in the 1975 film *One Flew Over the Cuckoo's Nest*. In the Academy Award-winning movie, Nicholson's character undergoes ECT, and his reaction shows a procedure that's horrendous.

I found something that offset the appalling association I had with ECT. A decade earlier, I read the book *Undercurrents*. The author, psychologist Dr. Martha Manning, fell into a depression so deep she opted for ECT. The treatments helped her enormously, and while she struggled with side effects of fatigue and short-term memory loss, she asserted she made a lifesaving choice. Dr. Manning's book moved me so much that I asked her if I could interview her for a *Fit* magazine article I was writing. The piece examined the effects exercise had upon women with depression. Ironically, when I interviewed Dr. Manning, I only asked her about exercise and depression because I never suspected I'd need, let alone demand, to have ECT.

Dr. Sylvia was the psychiatrist in charge of the Marine Parade's ECT program. When I discussed the procedure with him, I remembered Dr. Manning's transformational ECT experience. As scared as I was about the prospect of undergoing the procedure, I was comfortable with Dr. Sylvia. The physician, in his late sixties, had used ECT to treat his patients for years. There wasn't any pomposity about him, and he had an affable smile. A fellow coffee lover, he was never seen without a mug of Italian roast during his morning rounds.

"I want to do ECT. Please," I pleaded to Dr. Sylvia.

Dr. Sylvia made sure I understood the treatment's risks. But I didn't care about what could go wrong—I didn't care about anything anymore. Dr. Sylvia explained if I proceeded with the treatment, I'd have unilateral ECT rather than the bilateral version. The electrodes used to stimulate my brain would be placed on one side of my head instead of both sides. Unilateral ECT yields less intense side effects, such as reduced short-term memory loss. (Both unilateral and bilateral ECT creates a seizure in the whole of the brain.)

My ECT started at 6:00 a.m. and took place at the outpatient procedure unit. A hospital aide named Brian picked me up at the Marine Parade unit. I laid down on a gurney and was brought to the outpatient procedures unit. Brian had the perfect personality for such a job. Even though it was daybreak, he was personable and told me the ECT staff was excellent. Brian took me to a small, curtained room and Ellen, a clinical nurse specialist, arrived to prep me. She noticed I was trembling with anxiety and she reassured me I'd be in caring hands. Ellen gave my arm a squeeze of encouragement before saying, "Now, here's a little poke." I barely felt a pinch when she put a needle in my vein to start the I.V. line used to inject a muscle relaxant. I had never had a problem with needles or injections, and I was grateful that step didn't faze me!

At 6:10 a.m. Dr. Sylvia arrived, his coffee cup in hand. He wore a tweed jacket and tie, and he resembled an erudite college professor. Next, an extraordinarily handsome anesthesiologist joined us. Despite my severe depression, I couldn't help but wonder if my anesthesiologist moonlighted as a model. A small gas mask was placed over my nose, and I was eager for the oblivion that anesthesia would bring. As four staff members encircled me, my intense fear softened. Each person treated me with respect. They called me by my name and looked me in the eye. As Dr. Sylvia gently pressed several electrode pads on me including my scalp and temple, I could sense the medical team's compassion. No one harbored stigma in that room. These professionals chose this specialty because they wanted to help those who suffered from mental illness.

The anesthesiologist said softly, "Now, Dyane, I want you to count backward from 10."

I counted down to "5," then I was fast asleep. I didn't feel a thing. There was no pain at any time. When I woke up within an hour of the treatment, I was groggy, but I quickly became coherent. I had the appetite to eat a breakfast of scrambled eggs, toast, and orange juice that I had selected on a menu before my ECT. During the days following my initial treatment, my short-term memory loss was minimal. When I couldn't instantly recall something, it disturbed me, but the treatment's benefit was worth the unsettling temporary memory loss. I remained heartbroken over the loss of my father, but I no longer suffered from suicidal ideation. After I spent a week at the hospital, I was discharged and received additional treatments as an outpatient. Slowly but surely, my mood improved after each treatment.

ECT saved my life. The risks were completely worth it. I'd recommend ECT to those who feel acutely suicidal, to those who have been medication-resistant, and to anyone who needs to function as quickly as possible, i.e. a mother with young children or the breadwinner of the family. My health insurance covered some of the hospital costs, and I arranged an extended payment plan with the hospital for the remaining balance.

I learned of another procedure used to treat bipolar depression called transcranial magnetic stimulation, or TMS. TMS uses magnetic pulses to electrically stimulate nerve cells in the brain, and no anesthesia is required. Curious, I read Martha Rhodes' memoir *3,000 Pulses Later* about how TMS healed her major depression. TMS and ECT have comparable success rates, but there are some important distinctions between them. Currently, one must commit to almost daily TMS procedures for up to six weeks. TMS doesn't usually start working until midway through the four-to-six-week series. (ECT can cause depression to diminish much sooner, i.e. sometimes within the first few treatments.) However, a patient receiving TMS can drive back and forth to treatment alone. The hospital where I had ECT required patients to arrange a ride home after their appointments. This policy was, in part, created due to patients receiving general anesthesia. That rule created a major challenge for us. Craig needed to work and be the primary caregiver for the girls. We had no family members or friends willing or able to help get me to my outpatient treatments. But we considered my ECT to be a lifesaving treatment, and I needed it just like a cancer patient would want to complete the entire chemotherapy protocol, not just part of it. Dr. Sylvia strongly recommended I complete his recommended amount of treatments. On the nights before my ECT, we stayed at an inexpensive motel near the hospital. As soon as I completed the treatment, the four of us returned home.

Depending on one's situation, it would be worthwhile to examine the pros and cons of ECT and TMS before undergoing treatment, and research other treatments that have become available such as ketamine and deep brain stimulation. ECT is an enormous commitment, and it requires a profound leap of faith. It's expensive, even with health insurance, and TMS can also be costly. There are risks when receiving anesthesia, or when subjecting oneself to potential memory loss and other side effects. But despite the hardships and risks of ECT, getting the procedure done was the best decision I ever made.

CHAPTER TWENTY

My Booze and Benzo Downfall

I took an alprazolam pill, my first benzodiazepine, in the Marine Parade psychiatric unit. When the tranquilizer assimilated into my bloodstream, it eased my acute anxiety. Back then, I wasn't worried about becoming addicted to "benzos"—I only wanted to survive. After my discharge from the unit, I didn't become addicted to alprazolam, but several years later I turned to benzodiazepines when my anxiety became overwhelming. I promised myself I wouldn't become a benzodiazepine abuser, but once I took the pills, I was addicted before I realized it. It would take a traumatic wake-up call to convince me to give up tranquilizers forever.

I had always suffered from generalized anxiety, but my bipolar disorder intensified my apprehension, and each year it grew worse. When my angst reached its highest point, I called Dr. Arana and asked him for pharmaceutical help. He fit me into his schedule the following day and told me the majority of his patients took the potent, fast-acting benzodiazepine alprazolam. Dr. Arana wrote me a prescription for alprazolam, and after our session, I picked up the sedative at the pharmacy. I was deeply relieved to have the powerful pills at my disposal.

When I grew up in the 1970s, my father always had a bottle of the benzodiazepine diazepam sitting on top of his bureau, but I didn't know what it was or why he used it. Dr. Arana suggested I try the generic form of alprazolam instead of diazepam because it took effect more quickly and it was used to treat depression that accompanied anxiety. Alprazolam was also approved for panic disorder. Alprazolam didn't obliterate my anxiety, but it reduced its intensity.

Doctors typically prescribe benzodiazepines for a maximum of a few weeks for anxiety, but many psychiatrists prescribe them for months and sometimes years. Dr. Arana prescribed me benzodiazepines for months, and he never questioned my dependency upon the pills. I couldn't leave the house without my pills. One time when I forgot to order more alprazolam from my pharmacy, I was frantic. I called Dr. Arana so he could expedite the refill. When he didn't answer his phone, I left a series of agitated messages. I didn't calm down until he returned my call. After that had occurred, I timed my refill requests with military precision so I wouldn't run out of my pill supply again. Dr. Arana mentioned that most of his phone messages were from patients like me, desperate for our alprazolam refills. One of his patients wanted a quick benzo fix so badly, she lied to her pharmacist and pretended she was Dr. Arana to get a refill. While I'd never impersonate Dr. Arana, I understood the addictive mindset of his patient. During the time I took benzodiazepines, I didn't know someday my precious pills would stop working. I was unaware that after I stopped taking alprazolam, I'd experience awful withdrawal effects and my anxiety would increase.

It's common for people with bipolar disorder to "self-medicate" and use unhealthy substances and behaviors to cope with their distressing symptoms. As a teen, I despised alcoholism and drug addiction because I witnessed two cautionary tales: my father's alcoholism (used to self-medicate his bipolar disorder) and my first crush's cocaine addiction, which ruined his opportunity to attend college. But when my anxiety soared sky-high, and my depression hit rock bottom, I no longer judged substance abusers—I became one of them. The agony of bipolar disorder dominated my life, and I sought *anything* that would take the edge off my extreme anxiety. I self-medicated in vain. Not only did my anxiety return, I nearly destroyed the life of someone I loved.

A massive drawback of alprazolam was that it impaired my ability to drive. I caused two car accidents after I had taken my prescribed dose of alprazolam. One accident was minor, but the other one was much more serious. The first accident involved a church parking lot fence. I went to the church to meet with the minister, a kind man who had offered me the use of their meeting room for my bipolar support group. When I drove my car into the church parking lot, the alprazolam affected my depth perception, and I knocked down two planks of wood. When I told the minister I hit the fence, I felt guilty—it wasn't the ideal way to start our meeting! I didn't breathe a word about *why* I hit the fence. He would have every right to report me to the police for driving under the influence. The minister didn't suspect that anything was amiss, and he wasn't concerned about the small amount of damage. No one else questioned me about my fence "tap," and Craig fixed the fence a few days later. One would assume the fence mishap would be enough to convince me to taper off alprazolam, but I was in denial of the gravity of my problem.

My next accident was a nightmare that came close to being a tragedy. I had taken my alprazolam in the morning as usual. I took four-year-old Marilla to do an errand, and I secured her in her car seat in our Subaru Outback. Marilla dozed in her car seat while I waited at a stoplight and stared straight ahead. The light changed. I thought the light had turned green, so I entered the intersection, but the light had *not* turned green. Confused, I looked to my left to see a white SUV racing towards me. It was too late to put my car in reverse. The vehicle hit the driver's side of my car, missing Marilla by less than a couple feet.

An angel must have watched over us because no one was injured. We moved our damaged cars to an empty lot. An elderly husband and wife got out of their car, and I stepped out of the Subaru. Marilla, locked in her car seat, was now wide-awake and watched us without making a peep. I was in shock, and I lost control of my emotions. I bawled. What I had done was shockingly unethical. I was at fault, but the man's face looked guilty. He admitted he had been speeding, and said they were late for his wife's surgery. His wife got out of the car and gave me a hug, and I calmed down. Her husband didn't ask for my insurance information—I suggested we exchange phone numbers. I hastily wrote my information on a slip of paper and gave it to the driver. The couple didn't wait to give me their phone number. They jumped back in their car and headed for the hospital. I never heard from their insurance company.

After that accident, I tapered off alprazolam. Over a period of months, I followed *The Ashton Manual*, a benzodiazepine taper guide created by Dr. Heather Ashton and available for free on the internet. I pored over online discussions written by benzodiazepine addicts, and many of them claimed Dr. Ashton's advice worked for them. Quitting alprazolam was one of the toughest things I've ever done, but once I had placed other people in harm's way, I couldn't deny my problem.

I never got into an alcohol-related car accident, but as several more depressed-filled years passed by, my dependency upon it worsened. I traded one addiction for another and became a daytime drinker. I hated the taste of alcohol and I only drank it for its mind-numbing effect. In the mid-morning, I gulped a travel coffee mug's worth of cheap wine without tasting it. Afterward, I felt gross, nauseous and ashamed. I had transformed from being a health-conscious, certified personal trainer who only drank water to a depressed, overweight, anxious alcoholic.

Before I took tranylcypromine, an old-school antidepressant MAOI (monoamine oxidase inhibitor) in October 2013, I was advised to stop drinking alcohol. I was willing to quit drinking in a heartbeat if it meant I had the chance of wiping out my bipolar depression. On the day I filled my MAOI prescription, I quit drinking alcohol cold turkey. Incredibly, I didn't suffer from alcohol withdrawal symptoms, and I haven't had a drop of alcohol since then. I'd never tell anyone to stop drinking alcohol cold turkey because of the inherent risks. It's best to consult with a general physician or addiction specialist before making an extreme change. Groups with 12-step programs such as Alcoholics Anonymous and Drug Addicts Anonymous provide support for those who wish to cease their substance abuse.

Once in a while, I miss the anxiety relief that benzodiazepines and alcohol gave me, but I seldom think about these substances anymore. All it takes for me to stay off these addictive drugs is a glance at my daughters' faces. In less than a minute, I could've destroyed my life and Marilla's life because of my benzodiazepine addiction. In order to heal with bipolar disorder, it was essential to conquer my benzodiazepine and alcohol dependencies. If you find yourself stuck in the swamp of addiction, please help yourself and reach out for help. There's life beyond substance abuse, and apart from support groups, there are internet forums, books, low-cost therapists, and other resources you can turn to, some of which are outlined in Appendix D: Resources.

CHAPTER TWENTY-ONE

Disenchanted

Disenchantment, whether it is a minor disappointment or a major shock, is the signal that things are moving into transition in our lives.

—Sir William Throsby Bridges

After I had stopped taking bipolar medication and relapsed, I assumed I'd take lithium as long as my periodic blood tests showed it wasn't damaging my kidneys and other organs. Lithium kept me out of the manic state, but I remained depressed and lonely. I thought if I met mothers who had a mental illness, I'd feel less isolated with my pain. The thought of meeting moms with mood disorders gave me the strength to form a support group. I contacted the Depression and Bipolar Support Alliance (DBSA), a non-profit organization that sponsored support groups. DBSA required its support groups to affiliate with a chapter, but there were no chapters near me. I worked with their Chapter Coordinator to fill out the paperwork, and the Santa Cruz County DBSA Chapter was born. What was more daunting than completing the paperwork was the chapter's responsibility to pay yearly dues. I didn't have enough money to cover the cost, and I forgot to ask about scholarships, so I put my plan on hold.

October arrived, and the brisk air made me crave a chai latte from the Coffee 9 Cafe. While waiting for my drink, I checked out the community bulletin board and spotted an orange flyer advertising the annual Spooktacular Haunted House. The Spooktacular was a local attraction that had built up a devoted following over a decade. The founders were a community-minded couple that donated the admission fee proceeds to a different charity every year. I applied for the Spooktacular award, but I tried not to get my hopes up. When I was notified our chapter had been chosen, I felt a fleeting moment of happiness.

I met a kindred spirit at the first DBSA "Moms with Mood Disorders" support group. Sarah was the only mother I knew who had ECT for her bipolar disorder. Each of us had Dr. Sylvia administer our treatments, and I considered that a good omen. She understood the desperation that drove one to ask for ECT. Sarah was one of the few people in my life with whom I could be my true self.

On a January afternoon, Sarah and her five-year-old son Josh came to my house for a visit. After they had arrived, Josh glanced at me and smirked.

"You're fat!" he exclaimed.

My jaw dropped.

"Josh!" yelled Sarah. "Don't say that to Dyane—it's rude!"

Josh ran around our living room several times and leaped onto our old tan couch. He took off all his clothes, whooped with glee, and jumped off. Avonlea and Marilla screamed and sprinted into the other room.

"You're fat!" he repeated twice in a singsong voice.

No one had ever called me fat to my face! I was mortified. After they had left, I was tempted to gobble a pint of chocolate gelato, but when I approached the freezer, I stopped. Josh had done me a favor by breaking through the apathy caused by my depression. I was ready to stop eating a daily pint of gelato, and make some significant changes in my lifestyle.

As painful as it was to hear Josh's observation, he motivated me to take a step towards being healthier. I drank plenty of water each day. I had wanted to drink more water because of my lithium medication, which was a salt. Any psychiatrist worth his salt (pun intended!) would advise patients taking lithium to drink more water as long as it was a safe amount. When I spoke to Dr. Arana about water, he suggested visiting the Mayo Clinic's website to learn the most current recommendations for safe water intake. I drank a little over two liters (Two liters = 67.6 ounces) of water evenly divided over eight hours. Other people who drink this amount could get gravely ill. Drinking an unsafe amount of water can cause hyponatremia, a condition in which the level of sodium in one's bloodstream is too low, so it's essential to ask a trusted doctor about safe hydration before making changes. To spread out my water intake, I drank one 8-ounce glass each hour from 9:00 a.m. to 5:00 p.m. I programmed my cell phone's alarm for an hourly water reminder chime. I followed my schedule to the letter, for if I drank water past the early evening, it interfered with my sleep. Two liters of water is a large amount to ingest daily, and if I didn't keep track, I could easily drink too much. Therefore, I was careful. I rarely drank other beverages, and when I did, I reduced my water so I didn't exceed my limit.

An unusual domino effect took place. I suspected the amount of lithium in my system had decreased. Before I increased my water intake, I was always fatigued. (A side effect of lithium is fatigue.) Now I was more energetic than I had been in a long time. There was no other explanation for my increased energy. I didn't have my lithium blood level tested, so I can't be sure about what happened, but it was indisputable my fatigue had lessened a great deal. The water also helped my digestive system run smoothly. Even better, being well hydrated fostered a lightness of my body and spirit. I had been too depressed to contemplate exercising, but I was finally motivated to take a daily walk in the redwoods. I loved being outdoors again among the peaceful trees, and I walked while my girls were in preschool.

Next, I ate fewer calories and cleaned up my sugar-and-fat-laden diet. A few months later, Josh had no reason to call me fat. Even though my water intake, walking, and healthier diet improved my energy level and mood, my depression lingered. I obsessed about lithium's long-term effects upon my brain and other major organs. Once again, I believed I'd be able to think more clearly and eradicate my depression if I were medication-free.

During a get-together with Sarah, she mentioned the bestselling book *Anatomy of an Epidemic* by medical writer Robert Whitaker. Sarah's husband John had read it and found Whitaker's exposé fascinating and eye-opening. As a bibliophile, I was always on the lookout for unique books about mental health. My curiosity was piqued.

"Can you tell me any juicy details about *Anatomy of an Epidemic*?" I asked Sarah.

"I haven't read it yet, but John said he couldn't put it down. That's all I know," she said.

I requested Whitaker's book from the library and gave it no more thought until I picked it up. When I read *Anatomy of an Epidemic*, I let all my chores go by the wayside. The last time a book affected me so profoundly was twenty years earlier when I read John Robbins' classic *Diet for a New America*. Robbins' revolutionary book revealed harrowing truths about the meat industry. I became a vegetarian overnight. I found Whitaker's book extremely upsetting, for he uncovered disturbing, unethical actions within the pharmaceutical industry and the field of psychiatry. Whitaker examined Big Pharma companies' standard practice in which they frequently lied to the public. He uncovered medical studies that were designed by its authors and industry higher-ups to deceive people. These studies stated certain drugs as being the most effective substances when placebos were found to be more helpful. I had believed the results of some of those studies. Whitaker's book changed my opinion of the pharmaceutical industry. His message reached me because he seemed objective, and his extensive research backed up his statements.

I had entrusted the field of psychiatry and the drug corporations when I was at my most vulnerable. I naïvely thought all pharmaceutical company owners and shareholders wanted to help me. It was clear that many of these individuals cared more about money than about anything else. After I read about the controversial, Harvard-trained psychiatrist/author Dr. Peter Breggin I became even more disillusioned. He advocated replacing psychiatry's use of drugs and ECT with psychotherapy, education, and empathy. Dr. Breggin believed psychiatric drugs *caused* chemical imbalances in the brain instead of treating then, and he had a legion of devotees. I didn't subscribe to all his opinions, such as his anti-ECT stance, but I wondered if some of his assertions could be true.

It was unnerving and infuriating to discover that rich, greedy, powerful people were playing Russian roulette with our brains. After I read *Anatomy of an Epidemic*, I no longer trusted Big Pharma and psychiatry. Most significantly, Whitaker's findings inspired me to taper off bipolar medication again, but go about it differently and avoid a relapse.

CHAPTER TWENTY-TWO

When at First You Don't Succeed...

Before I had read *Anatomy of an Epidemic*, I was resigned to taking lithium indefinitely because it kept mania from destroying me. After I learned about Big Pharma's underbelly, I changed my opinion. Instead of regarding the medication as helpful, I turned lithium into the enemy. Demonizing medication was an example of the "all-or-nothing thinking" often done by people with depression. I thought I was less depressed because of a decrease of lithium in my system, but I wasn't sure. My overriding thought was that I couldn't return to a hopeless life. Only time would tell if tapering off lithium would eliminate my depression, or if I'd crash and burn.

Craig and Dr. Arana would be dead-set against a lithium taper because of the likelihood I'd relapse. I could never convey my perspective to them for they hadn't suffered from medication side effects or bipolar depression. I felt too fragile to confront Craig about wanting another shot at the med-free life. I ruminated about my situation during my walks in the woods.

I created a master plan based on deception. I wanted to prove I could be stable without lithium, but I wouldn't tell anyone I was off medication until three medication-free months had passed. At that point, I'd tell Craig the truth. Since Dr. Arana rarely required lithium blood level tests, it was unlikely my secret would be detected. My plan *seemed* like a good idea, but even if everything worked out, my deceit wouldn't sit well with Craig. I tried to ignore my guilt, but it returned again and again.

Sarah told me about Dr. Silver, her new psychiatrist who had an appealing treatment philosophy. She helped her patients take the least amount of medications at the lowest possible doses. I wanted to work with a progressive psychiatrist who I could trust. I called Dr. Silver to see if she would supervise my taper, and when we spoke, I didn't mention the deceptive aspect of my plan. Dr. Silver charged three hundred dollars for the first appointment, and she didn't accept my health insurance. I couldn't afford her fee. I had no savings, no credit cards, and I wasn't comfortable asking my friends or family members to borrow the money since I wouldn't be able to reveal why I needed it. I had a good credit score, but several banks turned me down for a loan because I co-owned our house, and my debt-to-income ratio was too high. I told Dr. Silver I'd call her back when I had the funds, but I had no idea how I'd make that happen.

During a walk, I glanced at my hand and noticed my wedding ring sparkling in the sunlight. *This ring could help me!* I thought. *I can always get another ring, but my sanity is more important than any piece of jewelry!* It wasn't a fancy ring, but I loved it. In a bittersweet, impulsive move, the following day I took my ring to a pawnshop where I barely got enough money to cover Dr. Silver's fee. I wasn't concerned Craig would notice my missing ring, but if he asked me where it was, I'd say it was getting resized. I was resolute about my mission, but no matter how much I rationalized it, I couldn't escape the ever-present guilt I felt about lying to my husband.

I was nervous driving to my appointment with Dr. Silver, but that was par for the course whenever I met psychiatrists. Her office was located in Aptos, a wealthy suburb. When Dr. Silver greeted me, she wore a hip St. John knit dress worth four or five of my wedding rings. I sat down on a velvet sofa in her waiting room to complete a health history questionnaire. Her office could pass for an opulent living room and had a fireplace, expensive-looking paintings and Eames office chairs. While she read my questionnaire, I took a moment to look at her more closely. Dr. Silver was attractive and wore tastefully applied make-up and elegant jewelry. I fiddled with my ring finger, which felt odd without its ring. After reviewing my forms, she looked up at me.

"Tell me more about your tapering plan," she said.

"Well, I'm determined to taper even though my husband is against it." I said.

"Pardon?" she said, her genial expression changing into one of dismay.

"My husband disagrees with my decision, but I'm going to do it." I said firmly.

"Unfortunately, I can't treat you if your husband is unaware of your situation," she said. I couldn't believe what I was hearing. Blood rushed to my face, and I felt faint. I had set my hopes so high that she'd supervise me, but upon hearing her words, they fell right down.

"Thanks," I mumbled. I was too upset and intimidated to ask for a refund. I stood on trembling legs and bolted out of the room.

My three hundred dollars, my wedding ring, and my expectations had gone down the drain. I was furious with myself for not telling the psychiatrist my secret before I made my appointment. While I was angry with Dr. Silver, there was nothing I could do. I would not breathe a word of this fiasco to anyone. I had to figure out another strategy. I didn't have more money to shop around for another psychiatrist. I was forced to brainstorm ways to convince Craig and Dr. Arana to accept my decision. I would have to be upfront—there was no other feasible option. I asked Craig to join me at my next session with Dr. Arana. When the three of us met, I announced I wanted to taper off lithium. Craig and Dr. Arana simultaneously objected, but I held up my hand and asked to speak for five uninterrupted minutes. They piped down, and I had the floor.

"Last time I stopped my meds, I didn't do a true taper—I didn't know *what* I was doing! I didn't do the right research. This time I have a plan. I'll do whatever it takes to prevent a relapse. I found out medical professionals recommend reducing the dosage as slowly as possible. One psychiatrist said to take three to twelve months to taper. I *know* it's an enormous decision, and I'm worried about relapsing, but I can do this!" I said.

"If Craig helps you, I can be a part of it," Dr. Arana said.

"I'll help her," Craig said. He looked at me, his face a mixed expression of concern, exasperation, and love.

Craig and Dr. Arana's skepticism only made me more determined to succeed. My desire to taper intensified after I watched an Emmy award-winning documentary by the British actor Stephen Fry. His acclaimed film *The Secret Life of the Manic Depressive* (available on YouTube) profiled people with bipolar disorder from all walks of life. Fry, a beloved mental health advocate, shared his bipolar experience. Out of everyone featured in Fry's documentary, only one person didn't take medication for bipolar disorder, and she was stable. Her name was Dr. Liz Miller.

Dr. Miller was the United Kingdom's first female neurosurgeon. In *The Secret Life of the Manic Depressive*, the attractive blonde-haired doctor discussed her life with bipolar disorder and her controversial choice to live medication-free. Dr. Miller changed her lifestyle and left the high-pressure world of surgery to become a part-time general physician She had been stable for a decade without medication. Dr. Miller and Fry were filmed strolling around a farmer's market where the radiant physician explained how she worked hard at maintaining a healthy life.

There's my role model, I thought. I'd do whatever I could to achieve long-term stability as Dr. Miller had done.

To taper, I needed to take my lithium in specific dosages that were unavailable by prescription. Craig extracted the lithium powder from my capsules. Using a high-precision digital scale to weigh the medication, he filled gelatin capsules with the amount of lithium I needed so I could lower the dosage bit by bit. Craig had experience using similar scales for his work, and I was lucky my husband was willing to do this task.

In December 2012, I was stable on only 300 mg of lithium per day. Soon it would be the Winter Solstice, a time of rebirth for many cultures. I chose that day to drop to 250 mg of lithium. The Solstice was also the end of the Mayan calendar. According to certain prophecies, the end of the world was fast approaching. Now that I had a goal, I wanted the world to go on! I prayed my taper would work. I wanted to serve as a role model to others. People were following my tapering journey near and far. I used Facebook and other social media to share updates on how I stood from week to week. All the while, I worried my plan would fall apart. The confidence I had felt when I made my decision to be med-free had subsided. I feared, *What if I relapse off lithium? What if I'm wrong and everyone tells me I told you so? What if I end up in the hospital? What if I feel suicidal? What if I let down my daughters and my husband?*

I resumed two activities for stress relief: exercise and reading. Sweating it out on my elliptical machine calmed my nerves. I visited The Icarus Project website, a resource for people tapering off psychiatric medication. The Icarus Project's success stories inspired and motivated me. I emailed Dr. Miller about my taper, and her encouraging response reiterated how she had tapered off lithium. Despite her positive example, I couldn't cease my pessimistic thoughts. I knew I was no Dr. Miller! I didn't have a medical degree, I wasn't a brilliant neurosurgeon, and I wasn't a co-star in an award-winning documentary. Comparing myself to her was like comparing rotten apples to ripe oranges.

When I felt dispirited, I wondered if my ECT and medications I had taken had damaged my brain. I countered my worry by reading compelling articles and medical studies about *neuroplasticity*, the brain's natural ability to form new connections to compensate for its injury. I liked to think that my brain was repairing itself! I searched for the latest positive psychology articles about how one's attitude could play a powerful role in one's health. Stories abounded in which doctors told their patients they had a certain amount of time to live. Their patients died exactly when the doctors predicted they'd die. I wondered if these vulnerable people had internalized their doctors' opinions to create self-fulfilling prophecies. Dr. Arana told me he never had a patient function without medication. There was no way I'd allow his words to sink into my subconscious if I could help it.

The day before the Winter Solstice, I walked at the high school track in the icy cold air. The bright sunshine and deep breathing revived me. I felt more hopeful, but I was anxious about reducing my lithium the next day. On the Solstice, a storm moved in and unleashed torrents of rain. I braved the downpour to visit a New Age store and bought two Reiki "energetically charged" candles designed to help a person achieve specific goals. I selected a crimson "Good Health" candle and a green "Manifest a Miracle" candle. Good health and miracles were exactly what I wanted. I intended to light the candles and say a positive affirmation as I took my 250 mg pill. While Craig didn't share my New Age enthusiasm, he took my simple ritual in stride, and the girls enjoyed blowing out the candles.

The Mayan prophecy didn't come to pass. The next day I woke up to a magnificent rosy sunrise with the Earth still intact. As the beautiful red-gold clouds disappeared, another storm moved in.

What will 2013 bring? I wondered. *Will I be able to prove I can be stable without lithium?*

As the New Year approached, I grew impatient and wanted to taper faster than I had planned, but I knew that was a very bad idea. I had to stick to my schedule. If I rushed the taper and relapsed, I'd never forgive myself. I was two months away from stopping lithium, and I was so close to my goal, yet it seemed maddeningly far away.

CHAPTER TWENTY-THREE

The Nadir

It was time for my counseling appointment with Ina, a mother I had met at the girls' cooperative preschool. A native German, Ina was tall with long honey blonde hair and pale blue eyes. In our brief interactions at the preschool, she was confident and serene. When I discovered what Ina did for a living, I was curious to see if we could work together.

One morning after I dropped off the girls at preschool, I returned to my car feeling dejected. As I sat in my Subaru, I was overcome by grief about my father's death, and tears spilled down my cheeks. At that moment, Ina walked past my car. I wiped my face and opened the door to run after her. When I caught up with Ina, I explained I needed a therapist. She agreed we could meet to see if she was a good fit.

During our first session, I described how bipolar disorder had affected my life and why I was tapering off lithium. Ina's insights were helpful, and her scholarly German accent was calming. I was relieved our time together wasn't completely serious—she had a great sense of humor. We kept our boundaries clear in public, and when I saw her at the preschool and the market, I didn't refer to our sessions.

After I had made another decrease in my lithium dosage, two weeks passed by without any problems. I wasn't hypomanic or acutely depressed, and I was cautiously optimistic. To stay motivated, I read books about natural healing for bipolar disorder while the girls attended preschool. At night, I read inspiring memoirs. I was drawn to accounts written by people with catastrophic diseases. I never got bored reading about the resiliency of the human spirit. When I read about someone who went into remission after battling a serious illness, I felt more optimistic. I wanted to learn how the authors attained such extraordinary healing. If someone else could go into remission, why couldn't I? Remission was my goal, although if a cure for bipolar disorder were found, I'd welcome it with open arms! It seemed plausible that our attitudes could make or break our health, but throughout my life, I couldn't summon a fighting spirit when something awful happened. It was all too easy for me to fall into apathy and despair.

To increase the odds of my taper's success, I recommitted to a health routine. I walked in the woods or worked out on my elliptical, I drank water, and I used my SunBox light in the morning for twenty minutes. The holistic bipolar books listed diet, not sleep, as the most critical factor for stability. A balanced diet *and* sleep were essential for health, but the holistic viewpoint drove me to eat healthier foods. While I preferred caffeine, chocolate, sugar, and cheese to tofu and quinoa, I resolved to work on eating better more than I ever had before. I checked out the latest nutrition books from the library and made small but significant changes such as reducing sugar and eating more organic vegetables. While I got my dietary act together I thought it would be wise to be extra-cautious, so I extended my taper to March 18, 2013, my forty-third birthday—the last day I'd take lithium.

The year 2012 had been a turning point in my life. I learned I could live without chronic depression clouding my days, and that was something I *never* thought would happen again. In our most recent session, Ina remarked that I had made great progress. I was thrilled to hear her clear-eyed observation, but she wasn't giving me permission to become complacent. Ina told me, "I think no one can be completely healed, Dyane—healing is an ongoing journey. Always remember that."

Ina's comment was profound. I'd need to remain dedicated to my health routine and monitor my bipolar disorder the rest of my life.

On the last afternoon of 2012, I used the elliptical trainer for forty-five minutes. I pushed myself on the machine because I felt the workouts strengthened my brain as well as my quadriceps muscles. January 1, 2013, marked the day I dropped to 150 mg of lithium. I was frustrated and impatient because many anecdotes I read described people who went off their drugs quickly or cold turkey without a hitch. But for every success, there were plenty of horror stories in which those who renounced their medications relapsed. Some people became psychotic and suicidal. I tried not to dwell on the dark side of giving up medication, but it wasn't easy for someone like me who ruminated about what could go wrong.

As soon as I got out of bed at dawn, I began my usual routine. I used my SunBox while the girls slept another hour. It was a very cold winter, so I exchanged my outdoor walk for an afternoon workout on the elliptical trainer. Later on, I felt unusually irritable and wondered if my mood had anything to do with my taper.

January 6 marked the fourth anniversary of my father's death. I thought about my father throughout the day. I silently implored his spirit to help me so I could be med-free, stable, and live a fulfilling life.

I was free from my all-consuming depression, but I remained anxious, frustrated, and sad. My temperament was changing. One night eight-year-old Avonlea accidentally rammed her knee into my stomach. While the bump hurt, my reaction was over the top. I yelled at her excessively, and my daughter's face crumpled. Avonlea began sobbing, and I felt awful. I apologized profusely, and she was quick to forgive me. Still, I lost my temper far too often with my loving, sensitive girls. In retrospect, what happened that night with Avonlea was a sign my brain chemistry was heading downhill.

Despite the stomach bump incident, Ina didn't consider me to be veering toward a crisis. I was astonished when she said we could tackle "regular" issues such as parenting and my marriage. While it was a relief to hear a professional say I wasn't in crisis mode, I feared it was only a matter of time before another disaster occurred. I suppressed my misgivings instead of bringing them up in therapy where they belonged.

When February arrived, I dropped to 125 mg of lithium and felt my energy shift into a higher gear. Craig noticed the difference. He was concerned, but we didn't think hypomania had set in. We were wrong.

Spring arrived, and Craig and I had our birthdays in late March. I enlisted Avonlea and Marilla to help me plan his surprise birthday party, and they had a blast picking out the decorations and his cake. In the past, my depression had prevented me from attending parties. The thought of hosting a celebration was unthinkable. The only reason I could pull off the event was due to my hypomania. I appeared to our guests as nothing but joyful—our children's happy faces and my husband's excitement were perfect reasons for my exuberance. No one thought I was about to skyrocket into mania.

In April, Craig and Ina noticed I was manic. I was spending too much money, acting hyper, talking almost nonstop, and exhibiting other symptoms of mania, such as barely sleeping. When the girls were at school, Craig and I argued about my wish to follow through with the taper. Every argument had the same script:

"Dyane, you need to stop this—you're acting manic," Craig said.

"There's no way in hell I'm stopping now—I'm too close to being med-free, and I'm doing fine!" I yelled at him, in complete denial of the truth.

"This tapering experiment is NOT working!" Craig yelled back in exasperation. Sobbing, I ran away and holed myself up in the bathroom.

In June I was down to only 25 mg of lithium a night, and my thoughts were racing. I couldn't ignore the mayhem in my head – I knew exactly what was wrong, but I didn't want to admit I was relapsing. I had tried so hard to make the taper work. As I realized my efforts were in vain, my depression returned with a vengeance. It wasn't ordinary bipolar depression, but the worst kind of depression possible: suicidal depression. Tears streamed down my face as I asked Craig to take me to the hospital. The moment was heartbreakingly familiar.

During the summer of 2013, I was hospitalized three times at the Marine Parade unit. Apart from Craig, the most supportive person in my life was Ina. She consciously, cautiously sidestepped the therapist/client boundary and invited Avonlea and Marilla to stay overnight at her house to play with her daughter. Ina kept in close contact with Craig about my situation and offered to visit me at the hospital. She lived two hours away from the unit, and I was deeply moved, but I didn't want Ina to make the long haul. I was ashamed of being depressed, and as much as I trusted Ina, I didn't want her to see me when I was so low. It would've been healing to sit with someone who cared about me, but I wanted to hide from the world.

That summer I found the drab, stuffy unit hadn't changed. I stayed at the unit three days and I resumed taking a large dose of lithium. But I was discharged too soon, and my suicidal ideation remained acute. In July I returned for a second, longer hospitalization, but after I had gone home, I was in terrible shape. Craig and I decided I'd return for a third hospitalization and we met with Dr. Sylvia about doing ECT again. Because of the severity of my case, I opted for the stronger bilateral form. When I received bilateral ECT, it helped bring me out of my suicidal state, which was no small thing, but my relentless depression remained.

My days at the unit were devoid of fresh air, outdoor walks, nature, or sunlight. No staff member had ever informed me about the hospital's policy of requiring a doctor's note to be brought outside for a walk. I would have recuperated faster and been less traumatized if I wasn't cooped up. When I left the unit, I swore it would be the last time I'd be a psychiatric patient. More than anything, I hoped that my suffocating depression would disappear.

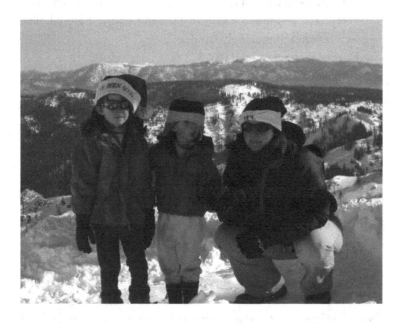

On vacation in beautiful Squaw Valley, California where I'm deeply depressed, and at my all-time heaviest weight.

CHAPTER TWENTY-FOUR

Redwood Baths and an Extraordinary Psychiatrist

When I returned home from the Marine Parade, life was drab and purposeless. The saving grace was the elimination of my acute suicidal ideation. The inpatient bilateral ECT I had done was invaluable in restoring my ability to function, but I wanted to participate in life, not merely survive it. Dr. Sylvia advised me to complete a round of outpatient ECT for the best possible outcome.

After the arduous summer, Craig didn't want to complain to me about his stress. At the end of each day, I noticed his tired, distressed face. His weary expression tugged at my heart, and I felt responsible for his fatigue and anxiety.

One evening I hugged him and asked, "Are you okay, sweetie?"

"I'm fine," he assured me, but I knew he was overwhelmed with taking care of our girls and keeping his geology business afloat. Before I relapsed, we struggled to keep up with our essential bills. My insurance didn't cover most of my summer hospitalization costs, and the amount we owed loomed over our heads. The payment plan I had arranged with the hospital would take us take a long time to pay off, but it was our only option.

Craig, drained by our family's needs, was daunted by the logistics of arranging my outpatient ECT treatment. No family members or friends could help us with my transportation. We couldn't afford to pay a caregiver to haul me back and forth to the time-consuming treatment sessions. As a bipolar medication-resistant patient, I was desperate to continue the bilateral treatments. I believed completing ECT was my only chance to alleviate my depression. After much deliberation, I made the controversial decision to drive myself to my appointments. Craig was skeptical of my plan and questioned me at length.

"Dyane, what if you black out, or can't remember where you're going?" he asked. I reminded him I had been completely alert after waking up from each bilateral ECT session, and I remained coherent the rest of the day.

At my last inpatient ECT treatment, I drew a giggle out of a nurse when I told her, "I feel like I drank a double espresso!" She and the other members of my medical team talked about how well I responded to the treatments. I took their observations into account when I spoke with Craig about commuting to my appointments.

"If I feel unsafe to drive, I won't get behind the wheel. There's no question about it—I'll call you," I promised.

Craig and I went to my first outpatient ECT appointment so he could watch me drive. Post-ECT, I was as careful a driver as I'd ever been during my two decades of driving. I was more alert than I had been in a long time. Craig agreed I was fully awake and responsive, and he confirmed that I drove safely. We felt we had done our due diligence regarding my driving.

Commuting to ECT was a grueling process. On treatment days my wristwatch alarm vibrated at 4:30 a.m. and I bolted upright in bed, wide-awake. (For anyone who has suffered bipolar depression, arising that early to make any journey is a major accomplishment!) The hospital required all ECT patients to arrive at 6:00 a.m. I quietly got dressed without disturbing the rest of the family and crept out the door when it was still dark and cold outside. There was never traffic at such an early hour. After I received ECT and woke up, I was fully cognizant of my recovery room surroundings. Post-treatment, I was hungry and devoured breakfast while a nurse took notes on my response to the ECT. All the while, I chomped at the bit to leave. After the nurses had observed me for a couple of hours, I was discharged so I could head back home.

Patients were instructed to arrange for a ride home after their procedure. I was extremely apprehensive about being caught lying to the staff. When I was told I was free to leave the hospital, a medical assistant asked me, "Is your ride here?" When I answered, "Oh yes, she's waiting for me in the parking lot," my anxiety soared. I wasn't caught, but I had some close calls. My intense fear and guilt over lying did nothing to help my recovery.

In retrospect, we could have used social media such as Facebook to put out a call for local help. We didn't know that using social media was an option. Nowadays it has become common for people faced with serious medical procedures to rally community support using the internet, and there are far more options available. Facebook has private neighborhood groups where one can post calls for medical help. Free virtual websites such as CaringBridge assist people with organizing medical logistics for patients and caregivers. Family members and friends can sign up on CaringBridge to offer help and receive updates. Other free resources for those facing medical crises include using local online parenting groups on Yahoo, and asking community newspapers to publicize a family's need for help. No family should ever handle medical treatment logistics alone.

In between my ECT appointments, I scraped by as a "minimum mom." On weekdays I helped Avonlea and Marilla get dressed and gave them cereal and other easy-to-prepare breakfasts. I dropped them off at their elementary school and headed back home until it was time to pick them up. As simple as the routine was, it took every ounce of my energy to get them ready and drive carefully back and forth to school. From the moment my eyes opened at daybreak, I was tired from the side effects of my medications, poor-quality sleep, and from depression itself. Navigating the aggressive parent drivers in the school's parking lot required me to be hyper-alert. I could have paid for the girls to take the school bus, but their bus stop was a dangerous spot on the highway, and the cost was steep. Most importantly, I wanted to be with my girls. Our drives to school gave me more time to talk with them.

Craig adjusted his work schedule so he could take Avonlea and Marilla to school when I was at the hospital for outpatient ECT. At home I kept busy doing the laundry, making the bed, and paying bills. To take my mind off my depression I read books, but reading was a temporary escape and I couldn't walk around glued to a novel all day. I had no desire to be with the few friends I had. Before I was diagnosed with postpartum bipolar, I listened to music, played my guitar, wrote in a journal, and talked with friends, but I no longer made any effort to bring fun and creativity into my life.

After completing my outpatient bilateral ECT, I wanted a fresh start with a new psychiatrist. I met Dr. Lath when I promoted the DBSA support group and posted flyers. I made the rounds of our town's office buildings, markets, and coffee shops, and one day I went to Dr. Lath's office building. As I entered the lobby, I noticed two men chatting and when they looked in my direction, I said "Hi!"

Dr. Lath glanced at my flyer and told me he was a psychiatrist. He asked a few logistical questions about the support group and I gave him a flyer. On my way out the door, I passed a coffee table covered with business cards. My eyes were drawn to a business card with the background of a rainbow and puffy white clouds. I did a double take and noticed it had Dr. Lath's name on it.

Wow! I thought. *What a cool business card!* I took a card from the stack in case someone in my support group needed a psychiatrist. It was the first time I had seen an optimistic-looking image on a psychiatrist's business card. The rainbow implied Dr. Lath was hopeful, and I sensed he was more compassionate than the average psychiatrist. When I wanted a new doctor, Dr. Lath came to mind. I called him and left a message explaining my situation as concisely as I could. Minutes later my phone rang, and I answered the call.

"Hi Dyane, it's Dr. Lath. I'm very sorry, but my practice is full," he said. I sat down on a chair, crestfallen.

"I've never begged a psychiatrist to take me on as a patient," I pleaded, my face flushing with anxiety. "But please, do you think we could meet? I feel like you could help me. The rainbow on your card...it's hopeful," I said.

There was a pause. I held my breath.

"Uh...all right, Dyane. I'll meet with you," he said. After having pushed myself so far out of my comfort zone, I felt a rush of relief and thanked him.

At our first appointment, Dr. Lath was warm and relaxed. There wasn't a touch of the arrogance, aloofness, or detachment that I had observed in other psychiatrists. Another benefit of working with Dr. Lath was his low fee.

"I'm curious—why is your fee so reasonable?" I asked.

He stifled a chuckle, and explained, "I want to make psychiatric care more affordable to those who need it." Here was a doctor who could charge twice his hourly amount, yet he was altruistic. It was refreshing. I was grateful to have a down-to-earth and kind psychiatrist.

Under Dr. Lath's supervision, I kept trying medication after medication, but I was still treatment-resistant. I didn't think any pill would ever help me, but I refused to admit it to Dr. Lath. At least he was willing to persevere to find a medication that would work. I continued taking lithium, and while it kept me from zooming into mania, it didn't reduce my depression. The daily 1200 mg of lithium I took caused my hands to shake. I couldn't apply eyeliner without zig-zagging the black pigment across my eyelid. The streaks I made on my eyes were appropriate for a Halloween costume or an Alice Cooper concert, not for everyday attire.

One morning while the girls were at school, I went to the library to pick up books I had requested. As I walked into the beautiful historic building, I recalled the last time I was there. I had visited the library months earlier when I was manic. I interacted with the staff without a shred of self-consciousness and enjoyed my visit. But on this day I was a different person who grappled with social anxiety and shame about having a severe mental illness. I kept my head hung low to avoid eye contact with the other patrons and staff. My shaky hands made it impossible to use the library's brand-new self-checkout system. Embarrassed, I walked over to Dale, one of the library's assistants.

"Hey Dale," I said as I gave him my library card. "Could you please help me check out these books? I'm having trouble."

"No problem," Dale assured me. I wanted to look into his eyes, but my anxiety prevented me. I was relieved Dale didn't press me to explain my absence over the summer. I had no idea what I'd say if he asked me where I had been. I scurried back home vowing never to return to the library unless I could check out books on my own.

The following day I met with Dr. Lath and sank into his office chair, quivering like an aspen tree in a storm. He took a measured breath before he spoke.

"Hi Dyane," he began, but I cut him off in a panic.

"Doctor Lath, look at this!" I lifted my hand, and it shook erratically.

"Why don't you drop to 900 milligrams a day of lithium. I'm sure the shaking will lessen," he advised.

We moved on to discuss another medication I hadn't tried: sertraline, a member of the SSRI family. Sertraline had been around for years, and my father had taken it, but it didn't improve his depression. I took 200 mg of sertraline a day, but it made me so tired I could barely get up in the morning. The medicine didn't touch the depression. When I informed Dr. Lath about my lack of a positive reaction, I cringed because I hated being a treatment-resistant patient. It wasn't my fault I didn't respond to sertraline, but I felt like a loser.

The lower dose of lithium decreased my shaking, but I wasn't free of all side effects. Each time I showered, handfuls of my long brown hair came out. I took the damp strands and spread them all over the shower wall. I had my reasons for doing such a weird thing—I didn't want all my hair clogging up the shower drain. But I also wanted my family to notice my hair loss so they'd feel sorry for me and give me attention. No one ever said a word about the hair on the wall, so I stopped my manipulative ploy and threw out the clumps after showering.

As the weeks passed, I experienced frequent flashbacks of being cooped up in the Marine Parade unit. I craved to be outside so I could feel sunlight on my skin and take deep breaths of fresh mountain air. Dr. Lath had encouraged me to walk for exercise again. Since my self-esteem was so low, I wanted a location where it would be unlikely for me to run into anyone I knew. I was blessed to live in an area renowned for its natural beauty. There were three parks located only minutes away from my house. I chose Fall Creek, an area containing twenty miles of hiking trails.

The first day I hiked at Fall Creek was a significant accomplishment. As I walked towards the woods, I stopped for a moment to take in my surroundings. Tears filled up my eyes as I acknowledged I had survived my illness. After having experienced weeks of breathing stale hospital air surrounded by other miserable patients, to stand outside in nature listening to birdsong was amazing.

Fall Creek is home to a centuries-old redwood grove. Hikers pass through imposing old-growth Douglas fir, Pacific madrone, oak, and ponderosa pines. When I entered the cool shade of the forest and sniffed the crisp, faintly spicy air, my hunched-up shoulders dropped to a comfortable position. I relaxed more when I heard the soothing, burbling sounds of Fall Creek. Glimmering rays of sunlight peeked through the tree branches. As I ambled along the path, I savored using all my senses in such a peaceful place. Although I was depressed, it helped to be around my "redwood therapists." The trees emanated a unique, nonjudgmental comfort.

I learned that being in the presence of trees has amazing benefits. In Japan, people practice *shinrin-yoku* or forest bathing, a practice recognized in their healthcare system. The term "forest bath" is intriguing, but misleading; shinrin-yoku means taking a leisurely walk among trees in which one aims to be present and notice the beautiful environment.

At first, my redwood strolls were quick showers rather than relaxing baths. I wasn't taking in my magnificent surroundings. Instead of gazing up at the ethereal shafts of daylight that peeped through the redwood branches, I stared at my feet. I ignored the refreshing, cool scent created by a combination of Fall Creek and the various trees' leaves. It took time to cease my habit of not being present, but after I read an article about the physical, spiritual, and emotional significance of forest baths, I was motivated to change my behavior. My love and admiration for the forest grew, and my walks energized and inspired me.

Studies have shown 20- to 30-minute-long forest baths are enough to reap health benefits. A 2010 study published in *Environmental Health and Preventative Medicine* found forest bathing lowers blood pressure, heart rate, and levels of the stress hormone cortisol. Some of the benefits are derived from the "bathers" inhaling the forest air. The trees emit organic compounds called phytoncides, and these substances are found in essential oils including grapefruit. The compounds not only protect the trees and plants from insects and disease—they can benefit people. A 2009 study published in the *International Journal of Immunopathology and Pharmacology* cited a link between inhaling phytoncides and an increase in the body's natural killer, or NK cells. NK cells, a major force in our immune systems, help identify and destroy infected, harmful cells. NK cells are considered important in the study of cancer. I read a summary of a 2007 *International Journal of Immunopathology and Pharmacology* study that stated forest bathing increased the activity of NK cells by an average of about 50 percent!

There was another convincing reason why forest baths could help anyone with depression and anxiety: the power of the color green. Color theory studies have verified that the color green triggers emotional responses including relaxation, calmness, happiness, comfort, peace, hope, and excitement. One reason the color green is thought to generate positive responses is due to our genetics; specifically, green environments signaled to our ancestors the presence of food, shelter, and water. I thought these studies and traditions were incredible, and it was validating to learn that my mellow walks had many health benefits.

With more than two thousand acres to explore at Fall Creek, I didn't come across anyone too often. As a woman walking there alone, there was a cause for concern about my safety. I bought pepper spray and reviewed how to use it. I always told Craig when I went to the park. He worried about me but he was glad I took pepper spray. When I walked, I held my spray in the "on" position, ready to use at any moment. I had cell phone reception deep in the forest, and I always brought my charged cell phone.

Apart from unsavory humans, mountain lions roamed the area, and there had been some recent sightings. My pepper spray wouldn't fend off an aggressive mountain lion, but attacks were rare. I read about what to do if I crossed paths with a mountain lion. The local UCSC Puma Project recommended, "In the rare event that you encounter a mountain lion, *do not run*; instead, face the animal, make noise and try to look bigger by waving your arms; throw rocks or other objects. If attacked, fight back." I wasn't overly concerned about running into mountain lions during the day.

As the mild Indian summer changed into colder weather, I wore a down jacket and thick gloves for my excursions. Despite my cozy gear, the walks became too chilly, so I used our home elliptical trainer. I missed Fall Creek's beauty, but at least the elliptical faced a window that overlooked redwood trees. I received a sprinkling of emails and phone calls from friends suggesting get-togethers, but my depression obliterated any desire to be social. Sarah was the only friend I wanted to spend time with, and I'm lucky I didn't burn her out with my dismal mood.

Apart from Ina, not a single friend or relative offered to visit me during the last three hospitalizations except for Craig and our girls. Granted, I realized not everyone in our circle knew I was in the hospital, such as my loyal friend Sharon who had moved to another state. It would've been helpful to create a phone/email tree before my health crisis occurred. Craig could have asked a friend to let others know of my whereabouts and suggest how they could help. I couldn't blame a friend who didn't call me if she was unaware I was hospitalized. But I harbored anger towards the people who knew my whereabouts, yet chose to do nothing. If I had cancer, a heart condition, or another less-stigmatized disease, I would've likely received visits, phone calls, and cards. Gestures of support, no matter how small, bring hospitalized patients comfort and remind them they haven't been forgotten.

The experience of being a mental hospital patient affects people in different ways. Some resilient souls carry on with their lives and don't dwell upon their hospitalization, but I wasn't one of them. After my seventh hospitalization, my generalized anxiety worsened, and I thought I suffered from post-traumatic shock disorder (PTSD) from the hospitalizations. I discussed hospitalization-induced PTSD with Ina. Although it wasn't her area of expertise, she concluded my theory was plausible. I knew it made sense to feel traumatized from spending so much time in a frightening, dehumanizing environment. I was determined to do everything I could to make sure I wouldn't return to a psychiatric unit unless I visited a patient.

In mid-September, I shuffled into Dr. Lath's office for my appointment. I wore my standard depression outfit: dark gray sweatpants, a nondescript black sweater, and no makeup. When I had been healthier, I wore jewelry, colorful clothes, and make-up, but these days I couldn't imagine doing anything more involved than applying lip balm. After I had sat down, I looked dejectedly at Dr. Lath.

"Hi Dyane!" he said in his usual cheerful manner. How I wished I could return his greeting with the same oomph. "How are you?" he asked.

"I'm still the same," I said. Dr. Lath sat quietly for a long moment, deep in thought. I could tell he was reviewing medication options in his head. I didn't leave him with many possibilities.

"I'd like to go ahead and have you take fluoxetine," he said. When I was Dr. Arana's patient, I tried fluoxetine, but I didn't respond to it and was puzzled by Dr. Lath's recommendation.

"Um, I tried it before." I said.

"Yes, I know you did, but I think it's worth one more try in addition to lithium, which you didn't take the last time you took fluoxetine. While some people with bipolar disorder can't tolerate the two medications together, they can be effective for others."

As soon as I left Dr. Lath's office, I drove to my pharmacy to fill the prescription for fluoxetine while I still had enough energy. I wanted to take my first pill as soon as I could. My rationale was the faster I got fluoxetine in my system, the faster I might feel relief. The following day I emailed Dr. Lath and wrote, "After our session, I felt a bit of hope—it was so great to feel that way again. You're doing a wonderful thing helping people like me!"

"Hope is the first sign of Recovery," was his brief, encouraging reply. *Please God*, I prayed. *Let it go right this time around!*

Unfortunately, it would go very wrong. The first time I tried fluoxetine, I had a neutral reaction, but this time fluoxetine gave me a skin-crawling sensation. The medication made me terribly agitated, and I couldn't sleep at night. I paced the living room at 3:00 a.m. I could only tolerate staying on fluoxetine for two weeks. Once again another medication had made me feel worse. I longed for the day when I could cast off the loathsome depression, but a loud, pessimistic voice in my head told me I was a lost cause.

I was thankful to Dr. Lath for doggedly suggesting medications I could try. Craig accompanied me to an appointment with Dr. Lath and touched upon Dr. Arana's shortcomings. Unbeknownst to me, Dr. Arana had complained to Craig about my failures to respond to medication. A wave of shame hit me. I had no idea Dr. Arana and Craig had that conversation. I felt betrayed by Dr. Arana for voicing I was a "problem patient" to my husband. I never wanted to try medication after medication! I never wanted to be a high-maintenance patient! Dr. Arana's disparaging, disloyal comments upset me, but his petty criticisms were in the past. What mattered now was that I had found a skilled, ethical psychiatrist on my side.

I continued doing what I could to feel better, which included walking and using my SunBox, but life remained bleak. I was trapped in depression's oppressive clutches, and while I couldn't imagine taking my life, I often wished I'd fall asleep and not wake up. It was no way to live, and my children deserved so much more than a despondent zombie for a mother.

In September 2013, after yet another trial of medication failed, Dr. Lath emailed me. It was the first time he used all-caps in his correspondence to stress his points. Since all-caps typically represents yelling or anger, I panicked at the sight of his message. Was he firing me as his patient?

Hi Dyane,

Thanks for your message. Summing up your situation, I can see that your mood disorder is going to be VERY challenging to treat. Please do not read this as me being less hopeful.

That said, given your lack of ANY seeming benefit from Prozac, etc., I think it's time to try something different. I don't really like switching meds by phone or email, but I want to now consider the monoamine oxidase inhibitors (MAOIs,) since they have shown robust activity, sometimes when others fail. There are other options (e.g. Latuda), but I'm also trying to work within cost limitations...

My best to you, Dr. Lath

It looked like I was in for another ride on the medication merry-go-round, and my hopes were as high as a snake's belly.

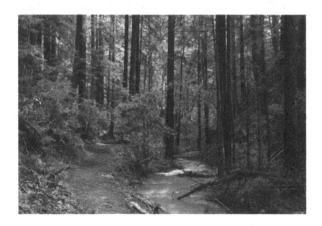

The peaceful grove where I took my redwood baths. Fall Creek, Felton, California.
(Photo courtesy of David Baselt)

CHAPTER TWENTY-FIVE

Holding My Breath

Where there is ruin, there is hope for a treasure.

—*Rumi*

When I read Dr. Lath's suggestion to try a MAOI, I was ambivalent. When I was a teenager, my father took a MAOI for his bipolar disorder. Dad's medicine didn't get a chance to do its job because he didn't comply with the MAOIs' dietary requirements. MAOIs have food and alcohol restrictions in which patients must avoid alcohol and abstain from foods high in tyramine, an amino acid. High-tyramine foods include aged cheeses, fermented products, and cured meats, products dear to many hearts including mine. If one is taking a MAOI and consumes too much tyramine, a hypertensive crisis can occur. Hypertension (elevated blood pressure) can harm one or more of the organ systems. Irreversible organ damage could set in with fatal consequences, so MAOIs are serious business.

Dad's MAOI experience didn't stop me from moving forward with Dr. Lath's idea. The bottom line was that I was willing to try any medication Dr. Lath suggested—I didn't care what it was, but as a jaded, medication-resistant patient, I had little hope for its success. None of my other psychiatrists had suggested the MAOI class of medication. I'd learn many doctors don't think their patients can follow and understand the dietary restrictions. I found their assumptions to be groundless because the majority of patients can handle the dietary requirements with proper guidance. I suspected another reason the MAOIs weren't often prescribed was due to the pharmaceutical industry. Pharmaceutical sales representatives have pressured psychiatrists to prescribe the latest, most expensive meds for their patients instead of the less expensive MAOIs that have been so effective they've been prescribed for decades.

Before I swallowed my first MAOI pill called tranylcypromine, I used the internet to learn more about the medication's history. What I discovered was encouraging and validating. I found a summary of a medical article confirming MAOIs as "particularly effective in the treatment of bipolar depression according to a recent retrospective analysis." The full version of the article appeared in a 2009 issue of the *Psychopharmacology Bulletin* and had an eye-grabbing title: "Revisiting the Effectiveness of Standard Antidepressants in Bipolar Disorder: Are Monoamine Oxidase Inhibitors Superior?" I couldn't access the complete article, but I wanted to learn more about this class of medication. I discovered on Wikipedia that MAOIs were known as the *"last-resort medication" for bipolar depression*. I was livid that none of my previous doctors had recommended a MAOI! I was so beside myself, I called Craig at his drilling site to vent my anger.

"Craig, get this," I said loudly so he'd hear me over the noisy chugging of the drill rig. "I'm reading about my new medication. It's known as the 'last-resort' for bipolar depression, well, except for ECT, I guess. Why the hell didn't the other shrinks mention it?"

"Honey, I'm right in the middle of a drilling snag, and the rig operator is acting like a jerk; let's talk about this later," he said, and hung up.

Tears formed in my eyes. By the tone of Craig's voice, I knew it was the wrong time to unleash my rage. I looked away from the computer screen, and a pang of deep loneliness hit me. I couldn't expect anyone else to erase my anguish. It wasn't reasonable to expect Craig to understand how I felt about incompetent psychiatrists. I promised myself I'd work on processing my pent-up fury with Ina instead of with my husband.

As I searched for more MAOI information, I learned that tranylcypromine was classified as a first-generation antidepressant. I located older studies that gave me cause for genuine hope. Patients with bipolar depression who took MAOIs with lithium were analyzed. In the book *Bipolar Disorder: A Clinician's Guide to Treatment Management* edited by Lakshmi N. Yatham and V. Kusumakar, the following section cites studies about combining tranylcypromine with lithium that yielded positive results.

> Four double-blind, controlled studies and three open-trial studies have examined the efficacy of monoamine oxidase inhibitors in the treatment of bipolar depression. In the benchmark study of Himmelhoch, Detre, Kupfer, Swartzburg, and Byck (1972), the authors demonstrated a 76% response rate to tranylcypromine in this subpopulation of bipolar depressed patients who were receiving lithium as well, and thus the improvement cannot be attributed solely to tranylcypromine.

I was astounded by the 76 percent response rate! I continued reading the rest of the section and learned that in a subsequent 1982 study by Himmelhoch, Fuchs, & Symonson, the authors examined 59 patients with anergic (a deficiency of energy) depression, of whom 29 patients had bipolar depression. A whopping 91 percent of patients on tranylcypromine responded compared with 24 percent on placebo. *That's an impressive result!* I thought. The response rate of the bipolar depressed patients who took a variety of MAOIs ranged from 53 percent to nearly 100 percent. Most of the studies used tranylcypromine successfully in the treatment of anergic bipolar depressed patients, and tranylcypromine demonstrated the highest response rate (81 percent) of any drug studied (Thase et al., 1992).

Other studies have been conducted on the effectiveness of MAOIs and bipolar depression. A 2015 study by Heijnen, Willemijn, De Fruyt, et al. titled "Efficacy of Tranylcypromine in Bipolar Depression: A Systematic Review" caught my eye. The authors wrote, "Currently, there is a paucity of treatment options with limited efficacy for bipolar depression. The monoamine oxidase inhibitor tranylcypromine might be an effective form of treatment." I wished the study also included lithium, but I was eager to read on. The study examined the effectiveness and safety of tranylcypromine in bipolar depression. There were 145 participants, and the response rates were higher in the patients who were treated with tranylcypromine. Participants had a 60.0 percent to 80.7 percent response rate with an overall response rate of 73.7 percent. Not bad! And those statistics were compared with placebo, imipramine, and lamotrigine. The *Journal of Clinical Psychopharmacology* reported the study's conclusion: "This systematic review provides evidence for the efficacy and safety of tranylcypromine treatment in bipolar depression. Additional research is required to establish the efficacy of tranylcypromine as an add-on to a mood stabilizer."

I was bleary-eyed after reviewing these studies, but I now had a sense of anticipation when I picked up the tranylcypromine at the pharmacy. The tablets were a Pepto Bismol-pink color—I wouldn't be surprised if they could glow in the dark. I swallowed the neon pill along with my daily 900 mg of lithium. Then I prayed. A flurry of negative thoughts followed my entreaties: *This won't work! These meds are a waste of time! You're a fool to think this will help!* Drained from my angst, I went to bed, eager for oblivion from reality.

October 2013 marked the beginning of my tranylcypromine/ lithium regimen. Within two days of taking tranylcypromine, I felt better.

Fittingly, my mood lifted on Halloween, my favorite holiday. To celebrate, I drove to my girls' school to watch them walk in the Halloween parade. If the parade had taken place two days earlier, I would've felt too depressed to leave the house, let alone face parents and teachers. I couldn't believe my depression was gone. I kept thinking I'd regress, and depression would envelop me. Over the next few weeks, I remained depression-free, but I didn't notice I was slowly becoming hypomanic.

On a warm afternoon, I drove Avonlea and Marilla to visit my friend Isla so we could tour her brand-new home. I had met Isla, a New Zealand expatriate, several years before I was diagnosed with postpartum bipolar, and she was familiar with my various moods. As I entered the foyer of the beautiful, spacious house, I spotted Isla, a shapely woman with short, spiky black hair and arresting light blue eyes.

I called out, "Hey there, Isla! Wow, I love your house! It's so huge. I can't believe it! You must miss the old one, but this place is in such a better neighborhood, isn't it? Is that a hot tub outside? Is that a pool? How fantastic!"

I had rattled off my greeting within thirty seconds, and I didn't give Isla the chance to get a word in edgewise. I was clueless I had abandoned the give-and-take of a normal conversation. Within a few days of my visit, I called and texted Isla several times, but she didn't respond promptly like she usually did. I had no idea I had turned her off with my rapid-fire speech and self-absorption.

My hypomania had been activated by the tranylcypromine, but it subsided a few weeks after I started the medication. Dr. Lath hadn't anticipated I'd become hypomanic since he thought tranylcypromine would be tempered by the lithium's mood-stabilizing effect. But our doctors can't always predict how the combination of these medications will play out in our brains. I was very thankful that my brain regulated itself. After the hypomania had disappeared, every afternoon I became much more tired than usual. Dr. Lath was unaware the tranylcypromine could cause fatigue. However, I read internet anecdotes that claimed tranylcypromine triggered fatigue. I didn't want to lower my tranylcypromine because it worked for depression. I held off on adjusting the medication and changed my schedule. I hoped that the fatigue would go away soon as some of the anecdotes claimed. After I picked up the girls from school, I rested for an hour. I resented the need to nap, but it was a necessary evil. When Avonlea and Marilla played near me, I stayed half-awake. If Craig was working from home, he took over childcare duty while I dozed. Over the next few weeks, my tiredness diminished.

Meanwhile, Isla returned my text, and we planned to meet over caramel lattes at Coffee Cat. When we got together, she shared her impression of my visit in her matter-of-fact matter.

"Aah yeah, to be totally upfront, it was hard for me to be around you. I was exhausted after our time together. You went on and on, you wally! I simply couldn't communicate with you," she said in her clipped Auckland accent.

While it was painful and embarrassing to hear about Isla's experience, I appreciated her honesty. I was grateful she gave our friendship another chance. We ended our coffee klatch with Isla giving me a hug, and my shameful feelings about my hypomanic ramble soon faded away.

As I continued taking tranylcypromine, I hardly thought about the foods and alcohol I wasn't allowed to have. Instead of moaning about how I couldn't eat blue cheese, I marveled at how much better I felt. I continued investigating MAOIs so I could get a reality-check about the often-maligned medication. Decades ago when MAOIs were introduced to the public, their risks weren't known. Because of ignorance, MAOIs had a reputation for being dangerous, and they were taken off the American market for a while. When MAOIs once again became available, they benefitted a countless number of people. As long as patients are under medical supervision, the MAOI drug class is useful for intermediate to long-term use. It's crucial to know besides the food and beverage restrictions, MAOIs can't be taken with many over-the-counter drugs, illegal drugs, prescription medications, or supplements. These limitations don't need to be a deal-breaker. When I've checked my MAOI's compatibility with another medication or supplement, I carefully read the medication's label. Next, I visit a reputable drug interaction checker website. If I'm still unsure, I call my pharmacist or email my psychiatrist.

While I missed eating foods I loved, tranylcypromine's benefit outweighed all else. At least I could enjoy my beloved chocolate and coffee in limited amounts. (Some doctors and organizations advise against consuming caffeine and chocolate while on MAOIs but Dr. Lath gave me the go-ahead. I've never had an adverse reaction to caffeine or chocolate.) Giving up alcohol cold turkey was challenging, but far easier than I expected it would be. As of this writing, I haven't touched alcohol in four years, and I feel much healthier ever since I became a teetotaler. Although tranylcypromine would be the missing link to lift my bipolar depression, my medications hadn't worked correctly yet. I'd face an agonizing medication-related setback in one of the most heavenly places on Earth.

CHAPTER TWENTY-SIX

Hell in Paradise

The mind is its own place, and in itself can make a heaven of hell,
a hell of heaven.

—John Milton, *Paradise Lost*

We planned to spend Thanksgiving in Kona, Hawaii. After postponing our vacation at Al's Kona Coffee Farm several times due to my hospitalizations, it was a highly anticipated trip. Al was a compassionate man, and he told Craig not to worry about rescheduling. When my tranylcypromine medication started working, we reserved Al's unit. Craig wanted to bring his mother's ashes to the Big Island so we could memorialize her there. She had lived in the Kona area for many years, and Craig thought Kona was the perfect place to honor her memory. I was filled with anticipation about visiting Hawaii, and I was eager to see our girls' reactions to the island's extraordinary beauty.

Two days before we boarded our plane to Hawaii, my depression returned. The situation was ironic, to say the least. I was bound for one of the most magnificent places on Earth, but I knew that wherever I went, I'd be stuck in a dark abyss in my mind. I searched the internet and found that some people took larger doses of tranylcypromine than what I took—up to twice as much. I called Dr. Lath and asked him if I could raise my dosage 10 mg for a total of 40 mg a day. He gave me his go-ahead and reminded me to be extra-cautious about how I reacted to the new dose. Negativity engulfed me, and I thought the increase would be a long shot.

During our flight, I enviously stared at the other passengers drinking mai tais topped with fresh purple orchids. We arrived at our Holualoa rental bedraggled and exhausted. Holualoa means "long sled run" in the Hawaiian language. Our lodging was on a steep mountainside in the middle of a thriving Kona coffee plantation. Despite drinking coffee for more than twenty years, I had never visited a coffee farm before.

As we unpacked our bags, the increase in the tranylcypromine made me feel much worse. I had insomnia and intense agitation in which I paced the living room from dusk until dawn. To make matters worse, as soon as the sun sank into the Pacific Ocean, eighteen wild Rio Grande turkeys gobbled loudly until sunrise. While their calls would've sounded cute during the day, at 2:00 a.m. the feral turkeys' trills made me want to feed them my tranylcypromine.

After two more tortuous days of taking 40 mg of tranylcypromine, my depression hadn't shifted, but my agitated insomnia worsened. I called Dr. Lath, and he advised me to return to 30 mg of tranylcypromine per day. I was profoundly disappointed with my brain chemistry. To plummet from joie de vivre to despair is the epitome of bipolar's cruelty. Most people would've been over the moon to be in Hawaii, but I couldn't get rid of my horrendous mood. I tried hiding my guilt, shame, and hopelessness to no avail. When we went on day-trips, I couldn't think of anything to say, so I remained silent for hours. I sat like a bump on a log while Craig entertained the girls with stories about his previous visits to the Big Island. Wretched, I felt my soul was gone.

When I spoke with Dr. Lath, he urged me to exercise daily despite how rotten I felt. I rolled my eyes in protest, but after I hung up, I dragged myself outside for a walk among the steep rows of coffee trees. I hated it. Reading a good book had been my way of coping with depressive spells, but my bibliotherapy no longer worked. I couldn't even focus enough to read. I wasn't motivated to visit a bookstore or read books on my Kindle. Apathy, depression's byproduct, prevented me from taking care of myself in ways that had previously helped me.

I attempted to self-medicate with food. On a humid, seventy-five-degree day, I wolfed down a large bag of local sweets called "Donkey Balls." The amusingly named macadamia nuts were coated with layers of milk and dark chocolate. The binge left me feeling nauseated and even more listless. I ate Kona coffee ice cream in a trance, not tasting any of the rich caramel flavor. I faced the inevitable sugar crash after each indulgence, and I wasn't doing my body any favors—I felt disgusting through and through.

During a few fleeting moments, the island's grandeur distracted me from my misery. We visited a breathtaking white sand beach in Kua Bay. Craig, Avonlea, and Marilla couldn't wait to swim in the gentle aquamarine waves. I watched my husband relax as he floated in the warm ocean, and I witnessed my girls' joy when they went boogie boarding for the first time. As I gazed at my family, a memory fluttered in my brain, reminding me of a time when I was depression-free. When I was fourteen, I went to Pacific Palisades' Will Rogers State Beach to boogie board in the cold water. The bracing sea's energy was exhilarating, and although I had goosebumps everywhere, I had the time of my life—wipeouts and all.

Now as I watched my family from afar, I was drained from my morose thoughts. How I wished I could be with them. Instead, I lay on the sand and people-watched, jealous of the beach-goers reading their books under bright-colored umbrellas.

We visited the town of Hilo twice during our stay. "Hilo" means "first night after the new moon" in Hawaiian, and Hilo soil is the official state soil of Hawaii. Years earlier I read articles about

Hilo's history of being struck by deadly tsunami. Ever since I was little, I was fascinated with tsunami, although I had never seen one. I had recurring tsunami nightmares. and asked my father if a tsunami could ever reach our home. He reminded me our house was high on the rim of a canyon, and assured me we'd be safe, but I didn't believe him. When I was older, I bought tsunami books and I watched documentaries about the catastrophic harbor waves. Once when I spoke with a man who believed in reincarnation, he suggested my tsunami obsession implied I had died in a tsunami in a past life!

Most of Hilo's beaches are nowhere as spectacular as the Big Island's West side beaches, but the water is inviting to visitors. We stopped at a pretty beach, but I had no desire to put on my shimmery blue Speedo swimsuit. I plopped down on the sand while the girls and Craig frolicked in the water. We were in the area where the devastating 1946 and 1960 Hilo tsunami had blasted inland, obliterating many lives within minutes. *Let a tsunami come and get me!* I thought. I doubted my depression would ever lift. But would I want my daughters and husband to suffer in such a disaster? Never!

I had known for many years that Hilo was home to the state-of-the-art Pacific Tsunami Museum. I never thought I'd get an opportunity to visit it, but my chance had arrived. During our first Hilo day-trip, I told Craig we didn't have to check out the museum.

"What?" he asked sharply. He didn't expect me to pass on visiting the museum. He knew it was exactly the kind of place I'd insist on visiting if I were depression-free. We both sighed in frustration as the girls begged us to stop at the Hawaiian Brain Freeze ice cream stand. I had a sudden burst of energy and grabbed hold of Craig's hand. I could do with a brain freeze to forget all my troubles, but in the meantime, I'd order a double scoop of Kona coffee.

When our family returned to Hilo a second time, we stopped at a small natural foods restaurant for lunch. As we sat at a window table with a view of downtown businesses, I heard cymbals clanging and drumming in the distance. The sounds came closer, growing louder until a group of beatific Hare Krishna disciples thundered past us singing "Hare Krishna" with gusto. The girls giggled as they watched the lively demonstration of faith. I hoped the rest of our meal would be quiet, but the Hare Krishnas returned even louder than before. They promenaded past us three more times, and proved to be a captivating sight to the other patrons, but I was so down that if a stark-naked Johnny Depp sauntered by, I wouldn't have peeked in his direction.

When our sandwiches arrived, Craig looked at my hangdog face and said, "You've traveled thousands of miles to get here. You've always wanted to visit the Pacific Tsunami Museum, Dyane. Now you're a three-minute walk from its front door! C'mon, let's go there!"

After lunch, I forced myself to visit a place I would've been thrilled to explore if I was free of melancholy. I thought the Pacific Tsunami Museum might be too scary for Avonlea and Marilla, but the front desk volunteers told us they had a section designed for children. An enthusiastic docent showed the girls their kid-friendly displays of earthquakes and waves. As the retired elementary school principal interacted with my daughters, I felt weary. I moved away from everyone and sat alone on a bench. I was embarrassed to be disinterested in a subject that had fascinated me for decades.

Each day in Hawaii I desperately hoped my depression would lift so I could feel some of the famous aloha spirit. While the word "aloha" is often used to mean "goodbye," "hello," and "I love you," there is a deeper meaning to the word. Aloha also means treating others with respect and being an engaged part of the world. I was full of anti-aloha sentiment, and I felt like an outcast in such a glorious setting.

Although Dr. Lath encouraged me to lower my caffeine consumption due to the tranylcypromine, I couldn't resist drinking plenty of the region's famous Kona coffee. High-quality Kona coffee costs at least $30 a pound. Once I sipped a cup of authentic Kona coffee, I understood why the pricey beans were in demand. When we arrived at Al's Coffee Farm, he gave us a pound of Al's Kona blend. The coffee tasted delicious, and I drank it daily, deep in denial that the caffeine contributed to my insomnia and anxiety.

During our trip, I was preoccupied with mortality, and with good reason. Craig had filled out the legal paperwork that allowed us to bring the container of his mother's cremains. We planned to scatter her ashes in a beautiful Hawaiian spot, and found the perfect place to memorialize her: a reef off the Puuhonua o Honaunau National Park. Also known as the Place of Refuge, this park was once the home of royalty and a place of protection for ancient Hawaiian lawbreakers. *Kapu*, or sacred laws, were the linchpin of Hawaiian culture, and the breaking of kapu could mean a death sentence. A kapu-breaker's only chance for survival was to make a journey to a puuhonua, or a sacred place of refuge. Once there, a forgiveness ceremony would occur, and the law-breaker could return to society.

The park was awe-inspiring. We took a brief tour with a park docent, and I was able to pay enough attention to learn about the area's sobering background of life, death, and freedom. The Place of Refuge had been a sanctuary to those who could reach it. Some people got so close to the border, but didn't make it. I wondered about what kinds of heartbreaking scenes had taken place where we stood. The scenario reminded me of Hilo: a place of natural beauty with a horror-filled past.

Craig found a small, inconspicuous beach next to the park. In search of a restroom, I left him with the girls for a few minutes. When I walked back to my family, I passed a huge plumeria bush.

I surreptitiously picked two handfuls of its creamy white- and orange-colored blooms. I handed the fragrant blossoms to Craig and sat down on my towel. He and the girls walked out onto the reef. There, they tossed the plumerias into the ocean as Craig spoke to the girls about their grandmother. After they returned, Craig decided it was best to scatter his mother's ashes by himself, and he went for a swim. He came back a short time later wiping his bloodshot eyes. Tears kept rolling down his face, and I gave him a hug.

I softly said, "I'm so sorry, honey, I love you," but I was detached. Depression often leads to self-absorption, and as I held my grieving husband in my arms, I thought, *I wish I were with his mom, wherever she is, instead of in this nightmare.*

A few days after we arrived back home, my insomnia worsened. I experienced two sleepless nights. I called Dr. Lath in a panic, and he prescribed quetiapine, a heavy-duty atypical antipsychotic with side effects such as weight gain, fatigue, and upset stomach. However, the quetiapine served as a lifesaver, for it nipped my insomnia in the bud. My nightly handwringing pacing was gone.

Then an even bigger miracle took place: my depression subsided a few days after I took quetiapine. The timing of the depression's remission suggested a connection between starting quetiapine and getting sleep, so I asked Dr. Lath if I could remain on a low dose of quetiapine. He agreed that would be worthwhile, so I continued taking the quetiapine over the next year despite its abhorrent side effects of fatigue, late-evening hunger, and a fifteen-pound weight gain.

Each morning after waking up I feared I had only been dreaming that my depression had gone. It took five minutes for reality to sink in that I was feeling better! I could laugh, feel hopeful, and write again, but it was never far from my mind that those blessings could disappear overnight. Apart from essentials known to promote mood stability (medication, sleep, exercise, healthy food, and counseling) what more could I do to prevent another relapse? The answer was clear—I had to research the latest findings in relapse prevention and do whatever I could to keep bipolar disorder from disrupting my stability.

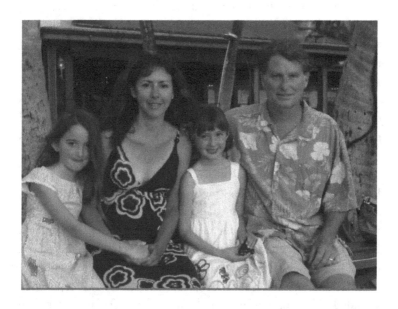

Depressed in paradise, Kona, Hawaii, November 2013

CHAPTER TWENTY-SEVEN

Never Be the Same

In the spring of 2015, I met with Ina for a therapy session. I was irritable and groggy from the quetiapine I had taken the previous night for insomnia. I had been stable and depression-free since we returned from Kona. Over the past year I had stopped taking quetiapine regularly, but if I couldn't sleep, I used it. I didn't want a bout of sleep deprivation to trigger hypomania. Even though it was hard to discuss my troubles, foibles, and fears with Ina, I valued therapy. I needed a safe place to unload and Ina helped me rise above my brain's negative chatter. I always felt better after we met.

"Ina, I'm sick of bipolar disorder. If it's not one problem, it's another. I wish I could rewind the last nine years and do it over without the bipolar horror show," I said.

"I want you to remember our mantra, Dyane—healing is an ongoing journey. There is no finish line," she said. I sighed. As much as I wanted to put bipolar disorder behind me, I couldn't. I needed to commit to what I *could* do: practice self-care (healthy habits), research innovations designed to promote mood stability, and if any of those new tools could help me, I'd give them a try.

When I was diagnosed with postpartum bipolar disorder, I was caught in a bewildering manic wipeout. I floated too high to be present with my family. When bipolar depression replaced mania, it contained aspects of the deadly tsunamis I feared since I was a little girl. The depression was a smothering force, annihilating what mattered most: my productivity, happiness, and hope.

I'd like to share what's helping me maintain mood stability today. Please keep in mind these are not one-size-fits-all recommendations. You don't have to overwhelm yourself with a complete lifestyle overhaul. Incorporating even one healthy habit into your life can activate profound change.

Life will always be demanding, and I'll never be exempt from challenges such as injuries, the death of loved ones, and grief. I'm always seeking what can increase my fortitude to help me endure painful times. I consider the search to be part of my "job"—the job of having bipolar disorder. I've found it to be hard work to accept the reality of the diagnosis and to monitor my brain. People with bipolar disorder who want a stable mood need to be vigilant in picking up medications, taking medications, handling health insurance, getting blood tests if needed, securing money to pay for these costs, etc. Some people can't take on all these responsibilities, and I'm one of them. At times I have to ask a family member, friend, professional or social services for logistical assistance instead of going it alone. One example is I have Craig pick up my meds at the pharmacy. It's a piece of cake for him, but I have social anxiety, and I never know when it will flare up. I don't find it easy asking for help, but I try to put aside my pride.

The foundation of my mood stability plan is a daily routine. On certain days I'm exhausted physically, mentally, or both, and I want to crawl into my bed and hide. But if I stick to my routine, I surprise myself and find the effort is worth it. Taking care of myself is empowering, and there's nothing indulgent or selfish about it. The more we practice self-care when life is relatively calm, the better equipped we'll be in facing difficulties or crises when they occur. Each person with bipolar disorder has a different list of helpful practices. These lists aren't set in stone. My list has changed over time, as will yours.

My Self-Care Habits (Daily unless otherwise specified)

- Alsuwaidan-Style exercise (See Appendix B for details/6 to 7 days per week)
- Medication
- Getting enough sleep
- Maintaining a structured schedule
- Meaningful work (volunteer or paid, schedule varies)
- Spending time with my family, my dog, friends
- Reading blogs, using social media (I take an annual social media hiatus for a few weeks—it always recharges me!)
- Supplements (Omega 3, Vitamin D3 and a B-Complex)
- Exposure to natural light, and in the fall/winter, my SunBox light
- Listening to music and reading
- Eating "clean" as much as possible, drinking lots of water
- Limit contact with toxic, negative, and draining people
- Write a blog post; blogging keeps me connected to virtual friends (weekly)
- Sessions with my psychiatrist (every eight weeks) and my therapist (biweekly)

Sleep, Exercise, and Medication

Sleep

Sleep is the linchpin to my mood stability. I prioritize sleep, but getting enough good quality sleep is difficult for many of us with bipolar disorder. As a parent of young children, my sleep is affected by my girls' occasional nightmares. The girls wake me up for comfort, which presents another challenge to getting a good night's sleep. (I'm hoping I'll sleep better when they get older!) Until then, I'm experimenting with MAOI-safe, sleep-promoting chamomile and passionflower teas. I want to try free and low-cost technological sleep enhancers such as the apps Relax Melodies, Pizizz Sleep, and Sleepmaker Rain, and any other safe sleep-inducing products I can find.

Exercise for Mood Stability: A Missing Link

My bipolar depression has made me want to do anything *but* exercise! Psychiatrist Dr. Mohammad Alsuwaidan changed my opinion about working out, and his guidelines have been profoundly helpful.

I listened to Dr. Alsuwaidan's webinar *Exercise for the Neurological Treatment of Mood Disorders*. Listen to the webinar at this link: kittomalley.com/2014/12/05/exercise-treatment-for-mood-disorders/

I had never been a webinar fan; it was too easy to get distracted and bored, but Dr. Alsuwaidan's webinar was engaging. He emphasized that exercise done according to his guidelines proved to be a missing link for his patients' mood stability. Once I heard his webinar, I considered my workouts to be one of my bipolar medications. Studies have confirmed that exercise helps depression, but there has been little compelling research done about how exercise affects bipolar disorder. Dr. Alsuwaidan emphasized exercise improved his patients' bipolar symptoms. Although he didn't have bipolar, he followed his exercise guidelines to keep his *brain* in good shape. I wanted to do what he did!

When I re-framed exercise as a mood elevator/stabilizer, I was motivated to work out. I wanted to follow Dr. Alsuwaidan's recommendations, so I read his article "Exercise and Mood Part Three—From Science to Action" (Appendix B: Dr. Alsuwaidan-Style Exercise includes this article.) I printed the article to review it with Craig, and he understood its significance. He was willing to watch our girls while I worked out and felt his additional childcare duty was worthwhile if exercise helped my mood stability.

Some days it's much harder to exercise, but when I consider bailing out, I think of this: within the *first two to five minutes* of walking or using my elliptical machine, my mood lifts, and my energy increases. I've been careful not to exercise on days when I have a bad cold, cough, stomach flu, or twisted ankle. I rest. I've had a few people call my daily routine "obsessive" or "compulsive," but they don't have bipolar disorder. They're usually coming from a place of concern, and I explain my rationale. If they can't be supportive, then I try my best to let their comments roll off my back.

A habit that helps facilitate my workouts is to put on exercise clothes and shoes an hour or so *before* my routine. If you work in an office or must attend a meeting, this won't be feasible, but getting on gear early has made me less likely to skip exercise.

I enjoy using mood-elevating orange essential oil during workouts. Before indoor exercise, I apply a few drops on my wrists' pulse points and the crooks of my elbows before an outdoor workout. Make sure to avoid exposing those areas to direct sunlight because essential oils can cause photosensitivity, and rashes can develop. Some people's skin can't tolerate undiluted ("neat") orange oil. If you have sensitive skin, add a few drops of orange oil to a carrier oil such as almond, grapeseed, or jojoba. Please do a skin test with orange oil if you haven't used it before.

Depending on the season, it might not be pleasant to exercise outdoors. Consider renting or purchasing a cardiovascular workout DVD for beginners that has reputable reviews. The key, as Dr. Alsuwaidan says in his webinar, is to break a sweat. Working out with a friend, attending a class, or walking your dog are great incentives and provides social stimulation. Once I began exercising for my brain's sake, I felt more empowered dealing with my bipolar disorder. It was validating when my daughters told me they noticed exercise improved my mood. They understand my workouts are "doctor's orders" and, for the most part, they respect my fitness time.

Life hasn't been easy since I committed to Dr. Alsuwaidan's exercise guidelines. I've had setbacks. A year ago, I felt moderately depressed due to situational events, and I was scared it would intensify. I was surprised when my depression receded quickly, and I think my workouts played a part in keeping the depression from taking over. I implore you to give this routine a try. Apart from taking medication, it feels awesome to do something that creates many positive "side effects."

Medication

Our brains have unpredictable responses to the mysterious chemicals we ingest. Each trial of medication seems like a game of Russian roulette. But give yourself the best possible chance to feel better. Work with an accommodating professional physician who will help you find a medication or medications to improve your life. It's essential to have a support system in place while you're trying new medications. Please don't go it alone because you deserve encouragement, love, and empathy. You may need to try different medications (a process that might seem almost as intimidating as climbing Mt. Everest), but you can do it.

I'm a proponent of old-school meds since they're responsible for stabilizing my mood, but new medications are being developed that are helping people. Some of these medications have given my friends excellent results, and they are worth serious consideration. If you can't afford the medication, ask your doctor for samples or find out if there are any low-cost programs sponsored by the manufacturer. You can contact the non-profit organizations listed in Appendix D: Resources for guidance. Above all else, keep trying, and don't consider yourself a "failure"—there are thousands of so-called "treatment- resistant" patients like you and me. If you've tried many medications to no avail, don't rule out options such as electroconvulsive therapy (ECT), transcranial magnetic stimulation (TMS), ketamine and others—you can discuss these possibilities with your doctor. At the time of this writing, there are new, advanced health modalities in the works, so I encourage you to research and discuss your findings with your doctor.

I hope a bipolar disorder cure will be discovered soon and make medications obsolete, but until that day arrives, please don't give up!

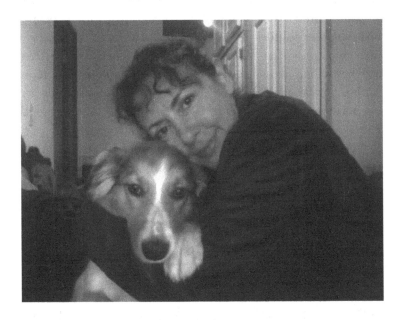

Spending time with Lucy, my "furry antidepressant."

CHAPTER TWENTY-EIGHT

Birth of a New Brain

It has been ten years since my postpartum bipolar disorder diagnosis. I wish I could tell you I've come to terms with having the mood disorder, but I have a ways to go. Despite being a mental health advocate, it's often difficult for me to tell people I have bipolar disorder because of stigma. However, our society's perception of bipolar disorder is improving. Recently the actress and bestselling author Carrie Fisher, one of the world's most famous bipolar advocates, passed away. She was honored for her extraordinary contributions to fighting stigma. The international outpouring of love and admiration for her was incredibly inspiring.

The mainstream media is making a greater effort to promote compassion and respect for those who have bipolar disorder. More celebrities are not only revealing their bipolar diagnoses to the public, they're serving as mental health advocates. Their powerful voices and large, loyal fan bases are helping diminish stigma. Mental illness anti-stigma campaigns are on the rise. A brilliant example is *Deconstructing Stigma: A Change in Thought Can Change a Life* at Boston Logan International Airport. The campaign was designed by the renowned Harvard Medical School's McLean Hospital and features the psychiatric nurse practitioner and mental health advocate Ann Preston Roselle. Ann lives with postpartum bipolar disorder. You can learn more about this courageous mother of three sons and her role in *Deconstructing Stigma* in the "Blogs by Moms with Postpartum Bipolar Disorder" section.

We can't predict when people who have bipolar disorder will receive as much empathy as people who have cancer or diabetes. Mental health advocates want to see bipolar disorder become a "casserole disease." We believe patients who suffer a psychiatric crisis deserve to receive casseroles, flowers, and cards like any other type of patient. I'm optimistic that people with mood disorders will be treated with greater dignity in the years to come.

While I support social media catchphrases such as #MoreThanADiagnosis and #imnotashamed, if I'm speaking with someone who harbors stigma, I backslide into shame. Feeling ashamed for having a brain disease is irrational; it's not my fault, but the shame is a deep-seated habit. During sessions with Ina, I'm working on how I can stop stigmatizing myself for having bipolar disorder. We've only just begun to focus on this issue together. I know there are role models who have bipolar disorder who have figured out how to let go of their self-loathing. Some of them are profiled in *bp Magazine* (listed in Appendix D: Resources section), and some of them are authors, entertainers, and people who live in my town. I plan on finding a few of these intrepid teachers, and I'm going to learn from them!

Authors have written bipolar self-help books promising readers they can beat bipolar, overcome it, or even be cured. As tempting as it may be to crush every bit of bipolar out of myself, I don't believe it's the most realistic, beneficial philosophy. Bipolar is a part of me and I can't pretend it's not there. On the other hand, I'm not advising that you befriend or love your bipolar disorder unless *you* wish to do so. We all have different opinions about our mood disorders, and our views about them fluctuate over time. In my support groups, I've seen women change from hating their bipolar to loving it (mania sometimes plays a role!) to accepting it as part of their unique personality.

Sometimes when I sink into a patch of mental quicksand, I share my challenges on my blog. (If the dilemma involves other people, I change the details and use fictitious names.) Most of my blogging friends have bipolar disorder, and these empathetic writers encourage and enlighten me through their comments.

If I don't feel like writing, I turn to other creature comforts. I use a bottle of mood-boosting orange essential oil (see Chapter Twenty-Seven for application suggestions), listen to anti-anxiety music on YouTube, take Rescue Remedy (see Appendix D: Resources for details), hang out with my dog, or watch a movie on Netflix. Some days I feel lousy no matter what I do, but it's worth trying at least one of these options.

There are free and low-cost mental health resources you can explore. (See Appendix D: Resources to learn about some incredible options.) If you need to talk, text, or chat online confidentially with someone about your bipolar and perinatal mental health challenges, there are understanding, trained volunteers and professionals available. In the app world, technologists have created recovery tools including the free apps Bipolar Disorder Connect, DBSA Wellness Tracker, and Moodlytics, and more apps are on the way. The International Bipolar Foundation and Postpartum Support International listed in Appendix D: Resources offer phone referrals, counseling, free online support groups, and many other services. Caring people run these organizations, and they're saving lives and generating hope.

These days I'm focusing on self-care techniques so I can be the most stable person I can be. To that end, I made a decision that didn't sit well with everyone in my world: I ceased contact with certain family members. My choice goes against the positive psychology movement based upon forgiveness as being healthy for the mind. Bipolar disorder is notorious for destroying relationships. While some relationships can be healed, my mood stability may be jeopardized if I remain in triggering, traumatic contact with some individuals.

After I was diagnosed with postpartum bipolar disorder, I assumed all my family members and friends would stand by my side during my struggle. I expected they'd offer to help me in small or more substantive ways. In previous years, I had helped all of them. When I became ill, some of my family members ignored me. I was shocked, heartbroken, and furious. To be shunned by one's flesh and blood while suffering from a mental illness has been an extremely bitter pill to swallow. In the rare event when they contact me, I don't respond. Instead, I turn to a self-care tool, I talk with my husband, or I meet with Ina to help lift me out of an anxious, angry state of mind.

As you can see, when it comes to forgiveness, I'm not a role model. I'm nowhere close to mending fences with those who let me down. On the other hand, when I realized I had to end toxic relationships and stop my people-pleasing behavior, I experienced significant relief. Nevertheless, I can't forget about these ravaged connections. How can I be the "most stable person I can be" when I can't condone family members for their damaging behavior? There's no easy answer. It's possible I'll forgive those who hurt me. What Ina told me bears repeating: "Healing is an ongoing journey," and as far as my inability to forgive is concerned, I'm at the beginning of my expedition.

Now I'm years away from my last hospitalization. I look back at the unforgettable phone call I made to my father about my diagnosis and pray I'll never receive the same news from my daughters. They know I have bipolar disorder, and they know it's a serious chronic illness.

"Mommy, will I ever get bipolar disorder?" my daughter Marilla asked me.

"My sweet girl. That's a good question. While there's a chance you could develop it, if you do, we'll know how to help you. Plus, there are researchers working hard to find a cure."

I felt compelled to tell Marilla the truth. I knew she wanted an honest answer, plus my precocious eight-year-old could tell when I was lying to her. If I fibbed, she'd see right through me. While I didn't want to give Marilla false hope, it would help her to know bipolar research is a priority for many scientists and a cure is possible. I wanted her to realize it's a manageable condition. My explanation assuaged Marilla's fears for the time being. Meanwhile, I hope neither she nor Avonlea will have bipolar disorder. I believe bipolar disorder can ignite creativity and generate other positive traits, but in my heart, I don't want my children suffering from this mental illness.

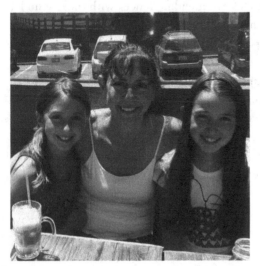

Dining with Avonlea and Marilla at The Cremer House, Felton, California, August 2016

When I think about the future of bipolar disorder treatment, it's anything but gloomy. As an International Society for Bipolar Disorders member, I'm notified about the numerous clinical trials that are underway, and about new treatment modalities that are in the works. Millions of dollars are donated to bipolar research every year. Advances in postpartum research include the amazing PPD ACT app that will help researchers understand the reasons some women suffer from postpartum depression and postpartum psychosis. The study will improve detection, prevention, and treatment of these conditions.

There's no way to sugarcoat the fact that bipolar disorder can feel like a soul-sucking tsunami. But you *can* achieve stability with this mood disorder. There are actions you can take that will boost your mood whether you're having a shaky moment or if you need to navigate a mental health emergency. Above all else, when life gets hard, don't give up! Reach out for support, whether it's to your friends, family, therapists, doctors, or a crisis hotline. (See Appendix D: Resources for crisis hotline information and non-crisis resources.)

Harvard-trained psychiatrist Dr. Shimi Kang, author of the bestselling book *The Dolphin Parent,* said, "Human neuroscience has shown that a mother's brain changes dramatically during her first pregnancy...One can say that a new mother has a different brain than before delivering her child." Since my brain was affected by pregnancy *and* bipolar disorder, my gray matter must be *very* different! But I'm grateful to my three pounds of neurons (the weight of an average human brain) for responding well to electroconvulsive treatments, lithium, tranylcypromine, and quetiapine. Sometimes I worry about my meds "pooping out"

(failing to work over the long-term), but there's nothing I can do about that. Besides, I can replace that fear with plenty of other concerns!

I feel good when I remember the other parts of my identity aside from the bipolar aspect. Once in a while, I like to pull out my dusty photo albums from my childhood and page through them. Other times I watch movies or listen to songs I loved as a child and teenager. I do these things because they remind me of who I am at my core. As powerful as bipolar disorder can be, it didn't destroy *me*.

I'm not reduced to a seven-letter word.

I'm much more than bipolar.

And so are you.

AFTERWORD

In her poignant memoir *A Circle of Quiet* Madeleine L'Engle wrote,

> *Because I was once a child, I am always a child. Because I was once a searching adolescent, given to moods and ecstasies, these are still part of me, and always will be. This doesn't mean I ought to be trapped or enclosed in any of these ages, the perpetual student, the delayed adolescent, the childish adult, but that they are in me to be drawn upon...my past is part of what makes the present Madeleine and must not be denied or rejected or forgotten.*

Just as Madeleine L'Engle didn't want to be trapped in a particular age, I don't want to be trapped or enclosed in a particular diagnosis. Bipolar disorder is a part of my life, and it may be a part of your life, but it's only a part. Our identities are as complex and mysterious as our Milky Way Galaxy. Thank goodness a single diagnosis can't define us, even though it may seem that way sometimes.

Indian summer has taken hold of the Santa Cruz Mountains I love. I bring my dog Lucy with me to walk in the woods and we pass a trio of Japanese maple trees. Their leaves are making their eye-catching transition from dark green to vivid orange. Next come the magnificent redwoods, the kings and queens of the forest. I breathe deeply, pleased with my newfound knowledge about the benefits of redwood baths. Lucy trots with a dolphin-like smile on her face, and wags her bushy tail with delight. When we come here, it's never far from my mind how glad I am to be in this sacred place.

I hop into my grimy white Subaru to pick up the girls after their first day of school. As I start the engine, a memory surfaces. I think about all the times I couldn't get out of my bed to take them to class.

"That can't happen again!" I whisper.

I drive towards the school and breathe shallowly. I'm no longer grounded in the moment. My fear of relapsing and returning to the psych unit has hit me hard. I'm aware I'm having an panic attack. I'm relieved I'm seconds away from the school parking lot and pull into a space. I stay seated and slowly, consciously breathe. I grab a homeopathic Rescue Remedy lozenge from my purse and savor its sweetness. It takes the edge off my anxiety.

I remind myself, *I'm here now. It's okay. I'm okay. I've been through worse. I can get through this.*

My fear recedes, and I'm able to draw a deep breath once more and carry on with my day. Getting through this attack is no small thing—it's a cause for celebration.

It's time to celebrate the birth of my new brain.

It's time to get to know my girls better, forest bathe, read, reconnect with my husband, create healthy friendships, laugh, and do much more.

It's time to stop always feeling that the other shoe is going to drop.

It's time for all of us with mood disorders to achieve our goals, whether it's getting out of bed at 6:00 a.m., taking on a volunteer job, or being present with our family. It's time to surround ourselves with people who love us.

In her transcendent memoir *An Unquiet Mind*, Dr. Kay Redfield Jamison wrote,

> *We all build internal sea walls to keep at bay the sadness of life and the often-overwhelming forces within our minds. In whatever way we do this—through love, work, family, faith, friends, denial, alcohol, drugs, or medication, we build these walls, stone by stone, over a lifetime.*

My wishes for you are:

- *Strength* so you may build internal sea walls using the healthiest of ways.
- *Support* when the sadness of life affects you.
- *Stability* so you may weather the overwhelming forces in your mind.

I hope the birth of *your* extraordinary brain will bring you much healing and happiness!

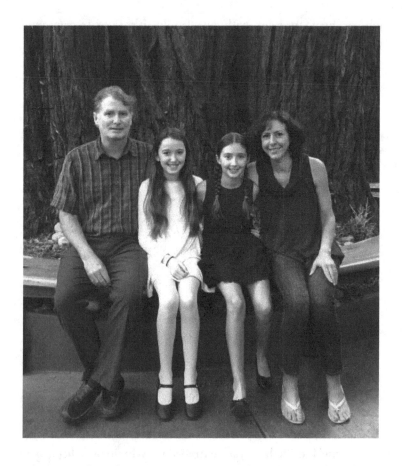

The Harwood Family, Casa Nostra, Ben Lomond, California, October 2016
(*Photo courtesy of Kevin Jandu*)

APPENDIX A

Postpartum Bipolar Disorder / Bipolar, Peripartum Onset 101

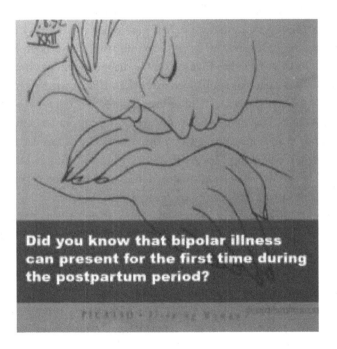

Did you know that bipolar illness can present for the first time during the postpartum period?

(Image courtesy of Karen Kleiman, The Postpartum Stress Center)

In the *Diagnostic and Statistical Manual of Mental Disorders (DSM-5)* postpartum bipolar disorder is described in the Specifiers for Bipolar and Related Disorders section as "peripartum onset."

This classification requires the onset of mood symptoms to occur during pregnancy or in the four weeks following delivery. (Note: The DSM-5 was published seven years after my postpartum bipolar diagnosis that occurred six weeks postpartum. The first four DSMs did not include a specifier for bipolar, peripartum onset.)

I asked a top perinatal psychiatrist and researcher Dr. Verinder Sharma if he could provide me with a statistic estimating how many women are affected by postpartum bipolar/bipolar, peripartum onset annually. Dr. Sharma's areas of research include neurobiology, treatment of bipolar disorder, and postpartum mood disorders. He has focused on the diagnosis and treatment of "subtle" bipolarity and published more than 100 papers in journals.

Dr. Sharma wrote, "Unfortunately we don't have the data to answer it. There are studies on the rates of recurrence during and after pregnancy, but data on the new-onset of bipolar mood episodes are lacking. Approximately 7.6% of women have an onset of a mood disorder (major depressive disorder or bipolar disorder) during pregnancy or postpartum (Viguera et al., *Am J Psych* 2011) however, it is unknown how many of these women have bipolar disorder. Another study reported the first onset of a depressive episode in 5.85% of women of which 15%-50% were later diagnosed with bipolar disorder. (Azorin et al., *Journal of Affect Disord* 2012). Dr. Munk-Olsen's research from Denmark has shown high rates of switching to bipolar disorder among women who have a psychiatric contact during the early postpartum period. Moreover, women with major depressive disorder are also at risk of developing bipolar disorder after childbirth. Thus, the peripartum period provides an excellent opportunity to identify women who are at risk of either first-onset or a recurrence of bipolar disorder."

In 2014 Dr. Sharma presented an outstanding webinar "Postpartum Management of Bipolar Disorder: Challenges and Opportunities" to the International Society of Bipolar Disorders.

I'm thrilled that there are physicians such as Dr. Sharma who understands the importance of researching and publishing about maternal mental health issues. I'm inspired by Dr. Sharma's mission to share with mothers on how they can best manage the onset of postpartum bipolar disorder.

There are six perinatal mood and anxiety disorders (PMADs) currently recognized by most perinatal specialists. Some PMADs share the same symptoms as other ones. The six primary PMADs are:

- Postpartum/postnatal depression (PPD or PND)
- Postpartum obsessive-compulsive disorder (OCD)
- Postpartum panic disorder
- Postpartum post-traumatic stress disorder/PTSD.
- Postpartum psychosis/PPP
- Postpartum Bipolar Disorder (Bipolar I or II, may be referred to as Bipolar Spectrum Disorder)

Postpartum psychosis and postpartum bipolar disorder often manifest together, but postpartum bipolar disorder is not always accompanied by postpartum psychosis. **To reiterate, postpartum bipolar disorder and postpartum psychosis are not always one and the same.** Some medical experts, websites, and articles state postpartum psychosis and postpartum bipolar disorder are the same PMAD. To make matters more confusing, there are medical professionals who maintain postpartum psychosis is part of the bipolar spectrum and experts who disagree with that hypothesis. This divisive issue is justification for further research about both PMADs so the relationship between bipolar disorder and postpartum psychosis is clearly delineated.

A 2013 CTVNews article titled "Baby Pinks? Postpartum Euphoria Can Be as Dangerous as Baby Blues" is one of the few mainstream articles to date that accurately and perceptively defines postpartum bipolar disorder. It contains an interview with Maya Hammer, a Toronto-based psychotherapist specializing in postpartum mental health. Hammer has worked with moms with postpartum hypomania and mania and observed, "In many women, the condition eventually clears up. But for others, it's the beginning of a long battle with postpartum bipolar disorder."

"Long battle" is an apt description of many postpartum bipolar disorder experiences. I found it validating to read "Baby Pinks?" since the media has rarely mentioned postpartum bipolar disorder, or if it has been brought up, it has been inaccurately defined.

There are bipolar and postpartum non-profit organizations that offer incredibly useful, often lifesaving resources. (Most of these resources are free.) I appreciate the volunteers and staff who make this help available. But some of the non-profits don't include postpartum bipolar disorder as a PMAD. Why? Ignorance plays a role along with the perception that postpartum bipolar disorder doesn't count as a bona fide mood disorder such as postpartum depression or postpartum anxiety.

The more awareness there is about postpartum bipolar disorder, the more likely a mother will receive the proper diagnosis and treatment. Accurate diagnosis is the most significant reason why it is imperative to know how postpartum bipolar differs from the other PMADs and other forms of bipolar disorder.

We all seek those who understand the type of life-threatening illness we've suffered. While I've had much in common with women who have experienced other perinatal mood and anxiety disorders (i.e. bipolar depression and postpartum depression have similar symptoms) postpartum bipolar disorder is a unique, complex set of symptoms. Each PMAD is a singular experience.

Until recently, I visited numerous PMAD and bipolar educational websites and I never saw postpartum bipolar mentioned. I became paranoid, and I thought my mood disorder wasn't considered valid by professionals despite being listed in the *Diagnostic and Statistical Manual of Mental Disorders (DSM-5)*. Even worse, I felt my PMAD wasn't worthy of support. My paranoia and frustration may seem irrational and a waste of energy, but if one hasn't suffered from postpartum bipolar disorder, it's impossible to understand what I call "the dilemma of omission."

I'm happy to say this dilemma is improving. In 2016 *The Huffington Post* published my article "Postpartum Bipolar Disorder—The Invisible Mood Disorder." The article contained quotes by acclaimed perinatal experts Dr. Shoshana Bennett (author of the bestselling *Beyond the Blues: A Guide to Understanding and Treating Prenatal and Postpartum Depression and Anxiety*) and U.K. obstetrician/perinatal mental health advocate Dr. Raja Gangopadhyay. The article was read by mothers, fathers, physicians, perinatal psychiatrists, bipolar and postpartum non-profits, and research organizations worldwide. It was wonderful to spread the word about postpartum bipolar disorder, and I've become confident about its rightful place among the other perinatal mood and anxiety disorders. In time, I believe more physicians, mental health professionals, postpartum and bipolar non-profit organizations, and others will recognize and provide education about postpartum bipolar disorder.

APPENDIX B

Alsuwaidan-Style Exercise

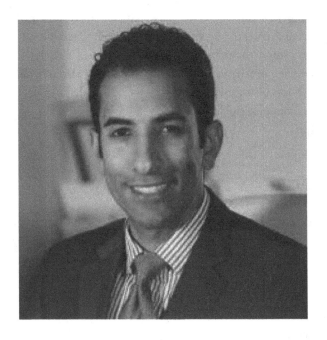

(*Photo courtesy of Mohammad Alshamali*)

In the following article, the psychiatrist Dr. Mohammad Alsuwaidan explains how to use exercise to achieve mood stability. I appreciate Dr. Alsuwaidan's down-to-earth, humorous, and wise "prescription."

"Exercise and Mood Part Three—From Science to Action" by Dr. Mohammad Alsuwaidan

How do we 'dose' exercise? What kind of exercise? What time should I exercise? For how long? How do I start and how do I keep going? For an easy reference, I will summarize the answer in one sentence then explain the details, and the fine-tuning will come later. Remember here we are talking about the 'dosing' of exercise that changes the biology of the brain and not the number of packs in your abs! (Although that might be a welcome side effect—if you are trying to achieve that, talk to a personal trainer.)

Here we are treating the brain and going after STABILITY! Exercise for 30 minutes, 6 days a week at a high-impact level. That's it! Simple, right? Okay, okay, I know it is not that easy. Let me explain further by breaking it down into 3 rules.

Rule #1

Exercise: For brain health, exercise can be any type that suits you. It does NOT have to be weightlifting or running on a treadmill. You do NOT have to go to a gym or use a workout DVD. Do any exercise you enjoy. Swim, run, hike, climb, lift weights, tennis, basketball, soccer, yoga, cycling, and on and on. Adapt the exercise to your body if your capacity is limited by physical needs or injuries.

Rule #2

30 minutes, 6 days a week: **The bottom-line is that the research shows this is the average of the dose needed for the brain to adapt**. Now let's break this rule down. First reactions from my patients are usually "6 days? That's a lot!" Yes, it

is, but we are only asking for 30 minutes. Think about it, how many hours a day do you use the internet or watch TV? Thirty minutes is very short. **In fact, DON'T do more than 30 minutes (unless you have a routine and have been doing this for years).** Doing more will lead to inconsistency and skipping workout days. The science shows it is far better (at least for the brain) to be consistent in exercising most days of the week rather than spending one hour exercising 2 or 3 days a week. In fact, for you gym-goers, if you think about it (and research also supports this) if you are spending more than 30 minutes at the gym then you're chatting and resting too much.

Thirty minutes makes it harder to come up with excuses such as *There is no time!* or *I'm too busy!* If you work often or travel, find 30 minutes to do some stretches, pushups, air-squats, jumping jacks, and so on. Thirty focused minutes is all you need. Done! Six days too much? Fine, 5 days is the absolute minimum, but better to aim for 6 so if you fall short then you have a day to save for later.

Rule # 3

High Impact: For the scientists reading this, that's 16 kcal/kg/ week. What? English, please! Here is how I explain high-impact to people: **For most of the 30 minutes you are exercising you should be sweating and it should be difficult to speak in complete sentences without needing to catch your breath. This means you work hard for 30 minutes, then you are done. Walking doesn't count unless it meets the criteria above.** Commuting does not count! That is your normal energy expenditure. Remember we are trying to change the brain, and you can't do that without effort.

Last Few Tips

- You can exercise anytime in the day that fits your schedule. I find first thing in the morning works best because it is the time of day with the least demands on your schedule. Plus, there is evidence this timing may have a more efficient effect than other timings. If it means you have to wake up 30 minutes earlier, then do it and go to sleep 30 minutes earlier at night. No big deal. But if it doesn't work, you can exercise at any time. That's the most important thing. Get it done.
- You can either start slow and build up to 6 days a week over a number of weeks or pick a week and start. If you have started and stopped exercise routines in the past, you will find this one is easier to maintain because it is more flexible. You can do anything as long as you break a sweat. Jumping rope is great if you don't have much equipment and can't go to a gym. Keep telling yourself it's only 30 minutes, and get up and do it.
- If you skip days and don't exercise at least 5 days a week, don't be discouraged and go back down to zero. Just start again. It is normal to stumble. I do all the time.

The important thing is to keep '30 minutes, 6 days a week' in your head and keep as close to that as you can. But the closer you are to that 'dose' the better the result will be.

At first, I followed Dr. Alsuwaidan's advice to the letter. But then my past exercise compulsiveness returned to haunt me.

I began overdoing it on my elliptical, and I eventually worked out twice as long as was recommended. I followed this "road to burnout" routine for months. Then I caught a cold and severe cough. Overnight, I stopped my daily workouts, and it took me more than *four months* to resume them. I knew I had to do something different to avoid a repeat pattern, so I chose an easier exercise that I could do with my dog Lucy. We took brisk walks so I'd break the sweat Dr. Alsuwaidan emphasized—no gentle rambles for us! I often got carried away and walked longer than thirty minutes. I needed to put the kibosh on that, and I did! As Dr. Alsuwaidan wrote, stumbling is part of the pattern, and it's only a matter of time before I'll stumble, but the important thing is to start again.

Dr. Mohammad Alsuwaidan is the Director of the Alsuwaidan Clinic in Kuwait. He was the assistant professor of psychiatry at Kuwait University and the University of Toronto. He trained in mood disorders at the Stanford University bipolar clinic and the Tufts Medical Center mood disorders clinic. He has received numerous awards and grants for his work including the American Psychiatric Association's (APA) Leadership Fellowship—considered one of the most prestigious resident fellowships in psychiatry. To read other articles by Dr. Alsuwaidan, please visit medium.com/@MoAlsuwaidan.

APPENDIX C

How to Create a Peer Support Group

I've found virtual support through bipolar-themed social media and blogs written by people with bipolar disorder. I've also yearned for real life encouragement, connection, and friendships with other women diagnosed with bipolar disorder, especially mothers. A peer support group can help you feel less isolated during your struggles. It's a unique chance to receive empathy from others who understand some of the challenges you face. Plus, if you create a women's support group, studies show being in the same room with other women raises levels of the "feel-good" hormone oxytocin produced in the hypothalamus!

When I first contemplated joining a support group, the closest meeting was an hour away, and I didn't have enough energy to drive there. I figured I'd wait for a group to form near my home or create a group, which seemed highly unlikely given the severity of my depression. After I felt better, I wanted to start a support group, but I made the error of taking on the project by myself. I'll come clean here: As a "control freak," I wanted to be in complete control of all decisions. I didn't want to coordinate or negotiate with another person. Being the sole facilitator would prove to be the main reason I burned out each time I started a support group. Hence, my #1 piece of advice is:

Find at least one person (someone with whom you can build good rapport) to help facilitate your support group!

Finding a co-facilitator might be a challenge. Ideas for your co-facilitator search include:

- Call or email your local NAMI (National Alliance on Mental Illness) or DBSA (Depression and Bipolar Support Alliance) chapter for referrals. Contact information for these organizations is in Appendix D: Resources.
- Call/email the closest mental health facility and contact the director by email or phone.
- If you have a therapist, ask her if she knows anyone who could help you.
- Send brief announcements to your local parenting and community websites, magazines and newspapers. If there's a fee, ask if it could be waived. One example: "Seeking co-facilitator for women's peer support group; contact (your email address) for information."

The Brass Tacks of Support Group Logistics

I had success in organizing groups and attracting members using the website Meetup at the cost of $15 a month. There can be multiple group organizers. As the monthly fee was a concern, I adjusted the Meetup group settings so members could contribute funds online. (Donations can be optional or a requirement, based on the setting you select. It's easier to do than it sounds here!) I brought a donation box to the meetings, and members usually donated enough money to cover that month's Meetup fee. The Meetup.com site will walk you through all the steps to form your group, in which you can create a name, description, add pictures, and so forth.

My Meetup group description mentioned the group was a peer-run group and not a substitute for therapy and medical advice. I advise that you do the same. You can search for other Meetup.com bipolar support groups for ideas about how to present your bipolar support group—there are all kinds, ranging from simple to more creative designs and text.

Once you've created your group's page, Meetup.com will promote it online. Your potential group members sign up for free on Meetup.com. They indicate all their group interests on a checklist, i.e. "bipolar," "mood disorder" and so on. When a Meetup group is created and tagged with any of those topics, the person is alerted by email. The group also appears in Meetup's new group section.

It's essential to make the group setting "private," which means only members can see one another's names, not the public. Some of your members will be extremely concerned about confidentiality. In the group description, be sure to state your group is confidential. If you have questions about privacy settings or want to double-check you did it correctly, email Meetup's customer service—they helped me make 100 percent sure the group was private.

Here are the bare bones logistics to plan and run your first support group's meeting.

1. Find and secure a good location/date/time. I decided we'd meet monthly. That frequency was realistic for my schedule and my energy level. We met on Saturday afternoon for 90 minutes, because that's when Craig could take care of our kids. We met in a yoga studio that donated the space. In the past, I've arranged with local churches and other non-profit community centers to use their meeting rooms for free. Libraries are worth checking out; they often have free community rooms you can reserve. Meeting directions were posted on our group's Meetup page.
2. Create a simple agenda to use on the meeting day.

3. Bring a sign-in sheet listing the following at the top: Date, Member Name, Phone Number, Email, and Permission to include a phone number and email for the group contact list. Bring pens.
4. Name tags = optional.
5. Cups, water/juice, and snacks = optional.

You can definitely create a group *without* using Meetup.com! Announce your gathering through submitting a brief description to your local papers' calendar sections. Make a simple flyer and distribute it to local libraries, coffee shops, and any other public bulletin boards. Find out what local mental health programs exist, including the closest hospital, and email them or send them a flyer.

At the first meeting, our members sat in a circle. I started on time and welcomed them. Looking at my notes, I reviewed a few basic ground rules. I reminded members the meeting was strictly confidential. Each woman had 3 to 5 minutes to introduce herself, and I used a timer to keep track, so no one spoke for too long. At the first few meetings we discussed a topic (i.e. "What's the number one thing that's helping your bipolar disorder?"), but then the group consensus was to change the format. At subsequent meetings, we each had the opportunity to check-in and talk about whatever was important to us. I set an alarm for ten minutes before the end of the meeting that reminded me to say we were near the end of our time together.

It takes a lot of work to create, promote, and facilitate a peer support group. Because I have social anxiety, it was a scary challenge to take on a leadership role. (That's a key reason why having a co-facilitator would have been helpful!) At least my efforts weren't made in vain—I found the support group to be helpful, and I even made a friend. I believe if you form a support group following these guidelines, you'll avoid burnout and enjoy the experience!

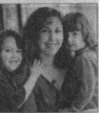

PRESS-BANNER

doesn't mean alone

A NEW DAY DAWNING

Dyane Harwood of Ben Lomond is on a mission to give support to those who don't often find it — women with bipolar disorder and depression.

NEWS. PAGE 7

Lucjan Szewczyk/Press-Banner

NEW HOPE: Dyane Harwood, shown with her daughters Avonlea (left) and Marilla (right), plans to start a support group for local women with bipolar disorder and depression.

At a glance

- **WHAT:** Peer support group for women with bipolar disorder or depression
- **WHEN:** 6 to 7 p.m., first Friday of each month
- **WHERE:** Mountain Community Resources, 6134 Highway 9, in Felton
- **INFO:** Dyane Harwood, 345-7190 or dyane

...bipolar disorder for much of his life.

"My dad was a gifted violinist in the Los Angeles Philharmonic for many years and lived an extremely functional life, some of the time," she said. "Growing up, I would notice that sometimes he would completely shut down, unable to leave his room."

Harwood said that her father was hospitalized many times and took numerous medications.

"Mental illness has the power to destroy a family,

just like any other physical illness," she said.

Many people who suffer from these diseases feel as if they cannot tell people in their workplace and personal lives or even some of their family members that they have bipolar disorder or depression, Harwood said.

She is determined to reduce the stigma of bipolar disorder and depression in her lifetime — one of her the reasons for starting the support group.

"There are women we encounter who seem like they are 'fine,' but they may be suffering from a mental illness and could use a confidential outlet like a support group," Harwood said. "I know this because I have been approached by some of them, and they are our neighbors and friends. I know that having a local support group for women can only be a positive element of our community."

Boulder Creek parent and

teacher Denise Schlaman, for one, is looking forward to attending.

"I hid my depression because it was 'shameful' and I should just 'snap out of it,'" Schlaman said.

Local professionals agree the group would be helpful.

"Women with these challenges can benefit greatly from a group like this," said Ann Andrews, a marriage and family therapist who lives in the San Lorenzo Valley. "They begin to realize they're not alone."

The group will meet the first Friday of each month at Mountain Community Resources Center. It will be a peer group with no professionals on hand to moderate, although a mental health therapist might join later to help moderate.

"I don't want these group meetings to be 'pity parties,'" Harwood said. "However, there will definitely be heavy emotions and themes discussed. My dream for this group is for our local women with bipolar and/or depression to feel less isolated and to help bolster one another with comfort, courage, inspiration and empathy."

Our local newspaper was happy to promote the support group.

(Photo courtesy of Lucjan Szewczyk/Press Banner)

APPENDIX D

Resources

If you're in the U.S. and thinking about suicide, please contact the National Suicide Prevention Lifeline toll-free at 1-800-273-TALK (8255) suicidepreventionlifeline.org—they are open 24 hours, 7 days a week. You'll be connected to a skilled, trained counselor at a crisis center in your area.

If you're outside the U.S., please visit this link for a list of international suicide hotlines: suicide.org/international-suicide-hotlines.html

The International Association for Suicide Prevention (IASP) has a database of international crisis centers at iasp.info/resources/Crisis_Centres/

Ashton Manual
benzo.org.uk/manual

The Ashton Manual is universally agreed to provide the best, most comprehensive information on benzodiazepine withdrawal. Professor Heather Ashton, DM, FRCP, is a retired British psychopharmacologist (an expert on psychiatric drugs) who ran a benzodiazepine withdrawal clinic in Newcastle, England from 1982 to 1994. Dr. Ashton helped more than 300 patients to withdraw from benzodiazepines. She's one of the world's foremost authorities on benzodiazepine addiction and recovery. This manual is an excellent resource for anyone beginning the process of withdrawal. Dr. Ashton recommends a very slow taper, which is what I did, and I had a successful outcome.

bp Magazine

bphope.com

For subscription questions call toll-free 1-877-575-4673

bp Magazine is the leading U.S magazine about bipolar disorder. Its tagline is "Hope and Harmony for People with Bipolar." Each issue contains articles, profiles of those living with bipolar disorder, and research updates. The *bp Magazine* website includes a blog by writers who have bipolar, caregivers, and medical experts. The website also has an online forum offering a variety of topics.

Crisis Plan Template and Guide

mentalhealthrecovery.com/info-center/crisis-plan/

It may sound intimidating, but I suggest making it a priority to write a basic psychiatric crisis plan to share with your family and the key professionals in your life such as your psychiatrist and therapist. If you're not sure what to write, ask one of your mental health team to help you, or visit mentalhealthrecovery.com/info-center/crisis-plan/ for a *free* crisis plan form.

It's well worth writing a plan to express how you'd like to be taken care of if you require a hospitalization. While it's advised to not write your plan in one sitting, it's always great to start the process. You can answer the easiest sections first and finish the other questions another time, perhaps with a support person to help you so you'll get it done as soon as possible.

Depression and Bipolar Support Alliance (DBSA)

dbsalliance.org

(Toll-free) 1-800-826-3632

DBSA is the foremost peer-directed national organization to focus on bipolar and depression. DBSA's mission is to "provide hope, help, support, and education to improve the lives of people who have mood disorders." The DBSA website's Peer Support section includes online peer support groups and an in-person, peer support group directory in the United States. The website has a variety of wellness tools designed for those who have bipolar or depression.

IMAlive Online Crisis Network

imalive.org

IMAlive is the world's first virtual crisis center where 100% of the volunteers are trained in crisis intervention. IMAlive's instant messaging/chat service is used to give people a safe place to go during moments of intense emotional pain. If you're in crisis or considering suicide, IMAlive offers live chat support with trained volunteers. It's a free, confidential service.

International Bipolar Foundation (IBPF)

ibpf.org

(858) 764-2496

The International Bipolar Foundation's mission is to "improve understanding and treatment of bipolar disorder through research; to promote care and support resources for individuals and caregivers; and to erase stigma through education." The website has a blog, webinar archives, and many other helpful resources, including the IBPF-produced book *Healthy Living with Bipolar* Disorder, available as a free PDF and geared towards the newly diagnosed.

International Society for Bipolar Disorders (ISBD)

isbd.org

(412) 624-4407

The International Society for Bipolar Disorders is the only bipolar-focused organization that shares emerging bipolar disorder research and clinical data with its membership. While there is an annual fee to join the organization, ask about scholarship memberships. The ISBD website presents outstanding webinars including one by Dr. Mohammad Alsuwaidan.

Marcé Society for Perinatal Mental Health

marcesociety.com

(615) 324-2362

The Marcé Society was named after Louis Victor Marcé, a French psychiatrist who wrote the first treatise entirely devoted to puerperal mental illness (puerperal: of or relating to a woman in childbirth) published in 1858. Marcé aims to promote, facilitate and communicate research about perinatal mental health. Members are primarily professionals; consumer members communicate with cutting-edge researchers in the field. There's an exclusive member electronic mailing list that shares discussions related to issues surrounding pregnancy and questions about treatment, medication, new studies, special cases, and more. The Marcé Society requires annual dues, but scholarships may be available; please inquire.

National Alliance on Mental Illness (NAMI)

nami.org

(Toll-free) 1-800-950-6264

NAMI is the largest grassroots mental health organization in the United States. NAMI's nationwide chapters offer in-person support groups for people with bipolar, their family members and caregivers. NAMI has educational programs designed to train people to become peer educators, a speakers' program in which NAMI volunteers visit public institutions to educate about mental illness, and much more.

Postpartum Progress

postpartumprogress.com

Postpartum Progress raises awareness, fights stigma, and provides peer support and programming to women with maternal mental illness. Their website has a blog and numerous helpful resources, including confidential chat rooms, for mothers living with perinatal mood and anxiety disorders.

Postpartum Support International

postpartum.net

PSI Warmline: (Toll-free) 1-800-944-4PPD (4773)

Postpartum Support International is my go-to website for the latest information about perinatal mood and anxiety disorders and support. The PSI Warmline helped me enormously. Dial extension 1 for Spanish and extension 2 for English. The Warmline messages are returned every day of the week. You're welcome to leave a confidential message anytime, and one of the Warmline volunteers will return your call as soon as possible, providing you with basic information, support, and resources in your area. If you're not able to talk when the volunteer calls you, you can arrange another time to connect.

PSI also hosts free, live phone sessions every week, including Wednesday chats for moms and **first Monday chats for dads.** During these sessions, you can connect with other moms and dads and talk with a PSI expert about resources, symptoms, options and general information about perinatal mood and anxiety disorders. The following PSI link lists U.S. intensive perinatal inpatient, outpatient, and partial hospitalization psychiatry treatment centers; check the PSI website for updates.

postpartum.net/professionals/intensive-perinatal-psych-treatment-in-the-us/

Rescue Remedy / Bach Flower Homeopathic Products

bachflower.com/rescue-plus/

I use homeopathic Rescue Remedy products for bouts of mild-to-intense anxiety. I've had people tell me homeopathic products don't work, or they poke fun at homeopathy, but since Rescue Remedy helps me, I ignore them! These products are safe to take with my MAOI medication; if you take medication, please check with your doctor or pharmacist to make sure there are no contraindications. I use Rescue Plus lozenges with vitamin B5 and vitamin B12, Rescue Pearls and Rescue Pastilles. Rescue Remedy is a blend of five different Bach flower remedies created by the British-born Dr. Edward Bach to be used during emergencies and crises. Rescue Remedy can be used for support with any stressful situations such as exam or interview nerves to the aftermath of an accident or bad news. Rescue Remedy was designed to help people (and pets!) relax, get focused, and become calmer. To learn about the exact content and the philosophy of Rescue Remedy, I encourage you to visit their website.

7 Cups of Tea

7cups.com

7 Cups of Tea is an incredible resource that offers free, anonymous, and confidential instant support through online text chat with trained "online active listeners" who come from all walks of life. The website offers online group support chat and a community forum. 7 Cups of Tea helps those who are going through a challenging time or who want to talk to someone.

People connect with listeners for different reasons, from existential thoughts to small, day-to-day things. A 7 Cups of Tea listener doesn't judge or try to solve problems and tell you what to do. They give you the space you need to help you clear your head. This service isn't designed for crisis situations, but the site offers a variety of helpful tools. Listeners who have bipolar disorder and who specialize in perinatal mood disorders are available for text chats. You can also pay it forward and become a trained listener!

RECOMMENDED READING

A *Mother's Climb Out of Darkness: A Story About Overcoming Postpartum Psychosis*, by Jennifer Hentz Moyer. (Praeclarus Press, 2014) Moyer's gripping memoir describes her suffering from postpartum psychosis when it was virtually unheard of in the United States. After Moyer was interviewed by *Glamour* magazine, her story made headlines, and she became an active advocate for women's perinatal health. In addition to postpartum psychosis, Moyer writes about how she was ultimately diagnosed with bipolar disorder, peripartum onset.

An Unquiet Mind: A Memoir of Moods and Madness, by Kay Redfield Jamison. (Vintage, 2009) If you're going to read only one memoir about bipolar disorder, select *An Unquiet Mind*. The extraordinary bestseller captures the experience of bipolar disorder in an eloquent, absorbing way, and it has inspired countless people. Dr. Jamison's book *Manic-Depressive Illness*, co-authored with the psychiatrist Frederick Goodwin, was first published in 1990 and it is considered a classic textbook on bipolar disorder. Following the publication of *An Unquiet Mind*, the clinical psychologist has been a prolific author. Dr. Jamison's insightful books cover topics such as exuberance, suicide, losing a partner, possessing artistic gifts and, most recently, the life of the poet Robert Lowell who had bipolar disorder.

Beyond the Blues: Understanding and Treating Prenatal and Postpartum Depression and Anxiety, by Shoshana Bennett and Pec Indman. (Untreed Reads, 2015) This book is the updated, bestselling classic from the highly acclaimed authors Dr. Bennett and Dr. Pec Indman. *Beyond the Blues* contains postpartum bipolar-related information. In the Perinatal Psychiatric Illness chapter, the story about "Tammy" mirrors my experience in several distinct ways as she was initially manic postpartum.

Death Grip: A Climber's Escape from Benzo Madness, by Matt Samet. (St. Martin's Press, 2013) When I suffered from benzodiazepine withdrawal, I came across Matt Samet's book, and the timing couldn't have been better. Of Samet's book, renowned benzodiazepine expert Dr. Heather Ashton wrote, "You do not have to be a rock climber to appreciate this book. Anyone who has experienced benzodiazepine addiction personally, or observed it in his family or friends, will find this book not only riveting but also helpful. Matt Samet tells his gripping story vividly, with anger and passion, and with no holds barred." Dr. Ashton's endorsement captures my enthusiasm for Samet's masterfully written book.

8 Keys to Mental Health Through Exercise, by Christina Hibbert. (W.W. Norton & Company, 2016) Dr. Hibbert, a fitness and postpartum expert, has written a unique book focusing solely on exercise for mental health. Moreover, she addresses pregnancy, postpartum mood disorders, and healing. Dr. Hibbert emphasizes it's not a workout or weight loss book, but "about teaching you the facts, skills, and tools you need to overcome your exercise roadblocks, become motivated, committed, and mentally stronger, and to flourish, reaping all the benefits exercise has to offer." Dr. Hibbert's positive attitude is reminiscent of Dr. Mohammad Alsuwaidan's philosophy regarding exercise for mood stability. This concise-yet-comprehensive book is a worthwhile read.

I'm Not Crazy Just Bipolar, by Wendy K. Williamson. (Wendy K. Williamson, 2014) In this bestselling memoir, Williamson candidly depicts her life with bipolar disorder. Williamson's raw, dark portrayal of her vicious depression is balanced by her remarkable sense of humor. Her introduction states, "I want you to know I am rooting for you. Yes, there will be ups and downs, mania and depression. Most of us suffer with these from time to time. Never forget there is peace too." Williamson's time-tested advice on how to weather the storms of bipolar disorder will benefit any reader.

No Wonder My Parents Drank: Tales from a Stand-Up Dad, by Jay Mohr. (Simon & Schuster, 2010) Jay Mohr is known as a first-rate comedian, actor, producer, and host of the cutting-edge podcast "Mohr Stories." His debut book *Gasping for Airtime* (a chronicle of his struggle with panic attacks and his years as a *Saturday Night Live* featured cast member) was a bestseller. Mohr is also a fiercely loving, hands-on father. In *No Wonder My Parents Drank,* he weaves humor, heartache and profound insights gained through a harrowing battle with male infertility and the agony of his son's premature birth. Mohr perfectly depicts the feeling of watching your child grow up: "As he grows, my heart sinks. The less he needs me, the more I need him." Mohr's stories of his vulnerabilities and triumphs as a father will stay with you long after you read this poignant book.

Preventing Bipolar Relapse: A Lifestyle Program to Help You Maintain a Balanced Mood and Live Well, by Ruth C. White. (New Harbinger Publications, 2014) Dr. White, an expert on bipolar and co-author of *Bipolar 101*, has firsthand experience with the mood disorder. *Preventing Bipolar Relapse* is the first book written that focuses 100% on the prevention of relapse. Dr. White's unique program SNAP (Sleep, Nutrition, Activity, and People) will help you avoid relapse. Dr. White also offers practical tips and tracking tools in this one-of-a-kind book.

Stand and Deliver, by Adam Ant. (Sidgwick & Jackson Ltd, 2007) London-born Stuart Goddard transformed himself into the world-famous musician Adam Ant. (Yes, one of my favorites!) He battled bipolar disorder in the public eye, and after years of illness, Adam Ant returned to the music world as a stable, productive and brave singer/songwriter. The musician's moving, fascinating memoir thoughtfully examines his remarkable life from pop star to an influential mental health advocate.

The Dolphin Parent: A Guide to Raising Healthy, Happy and Self-Motivated Kids, by Shimi Kang. (TarcherPerigree, 2014) Dr. Kang is an inspiring Harvard-trained psychiatrist and an expert in human motivation. She researched neuroscience and behavioral studies to reveal why aggressive "tiger parents" and permissive "jellyfish parents" can damage self-motivation. I love that Dr. Kang chose the intelligent, joyful, playful, highly social dolphin as a parenting model. Dolphin parents bring balance into their children's lives and guide them without being overbearing so they can be happy and healthy—no offense to tigers and jellyfish, but I want to be a dolphin parent!

The Midnight Disease: The Drive to Write, Writer's Block and the Creative Brain, by Alice W. Flaherty. (Mariner Books, 2005) In this book, the groundbreaking neurologist Dr. Flaherty explores the mysteries of literary creativity: what sparks the drive to write and what extinguishes it. She mentions intriguing examples from medical case studies and the lives of writers such as Franz Kafka, Anne Lamott, Sylvia Plath, and Stephen King. Dr. Flaherty, who disclosed her diagnosis of bipolar disorder after the publication of *The Midnight Disease*, grappled with episodes of hypergraphia (compulsive writing) and writer's block. Here she offers a compelling personal account of her experiences with these conditions. Dr. Flaherty's colleague, the author Dr. Kay Redfield Jamison, calls *The Midnight Disease*, "An original, fascinating and beautifully written reckoning... of that great human passion: to write."

The Modern Management of Perinatal Psychiatry, by Carol Henshaw, John Cox and Joanne Barton. (RCPsych Publications, 2009) This outstanding book provides a comprehensive overview of mental health problems associated with pregnancy and the year after delivery. Key topics covered include issues for children and families; screening for and prevention of mental disorders about childbirth; prescribing in pregnancy and lactation; and transcultural issues. Although geared for perinatal mental health professionals, it provides a wealth of information useful to all readers interested in maternal mental health.

Dr. Henshaw has been President of the Marcé Society for Perinatal Mental Health, a scientific society devoted to mental illness related to childbearing. She has served on the Executive Committee of the Royal College of Psychiatrists' Perinatal Section. Dr. John Cox has held the positions of President of The Marcé Society and President of the Royal College of Psychiatrists. A developer of the world-renowned Edinburgh Postnatal Depression Scale, he has more than 30 years of clinical and research experience in perinatal psychiatry. Dr. Barton is a Child and Adolescent Psychiatrist who works for North Staffordshire Combined Healthcare NHS Trust, providing psychiatric input to a community-based child and adolescent mental health service.

The Other Side of Silence: A Psychiatrist's Memoir of Depression, by Linda Gask. (Summersdale, 2016) Dr. Gask has a spare-yet-revealing way of writing about her innermost feelings, and her book has touched many people suffering from depression. The psychiatrist has firsthand experience of both pharmacological and psychological treatments for depression. Dr. Gask was born to a Scottish mother and English father and brought up on the east coast of England. In sharing her personal journey with recurring, severe depression and her successful treatment, Dr. Gask offers the reader hope. Dr. Gask is now Emerita Professor of Primary Care Psychiatry at the University of Manchester and is semi-retired. Visit Dr. Gask's blog about mental health at lindagask.com.

Two Bipolar Chicks' Guide to Survival: Tips for Living with Bipolar Disorder, by Wendy K. Williamson and Honora Rose. (Post Hill Press, 2014) The authors know this topic intimately as they both live with bipolar disorder. Williamson and Rose provide the latest strategies to cope with bipolar, and they incorporate humor when appropriate. The book covers all kinds of tools one can use to improve chances for recovery and stability. Standout sections include Chapter 11, "Treatments and Therapies," which reviews cutting-edge treatment possibilities and Chapter 9, "Sunshine," which contains suggestions I've found to be life-changing. *Two Bipolar Chicks' Guide to Survival* is the book I wish I had on hand after I was diagnosed with bipolar disorder.

Undercurrents: A Life Beneath the Surface, by Martha Manning. (Harper One, 1995) Dr. Manning's book influenced me about the benefits of electroconvulsive therapy (ECT) long before I elected to have the procedure done. Dr. Manning, a clinical psychologist, wife, and mother, experienced debilitating depression. She tried medications and psychiatric counseling but remained extremely depressed. ECT helped bring her out of her suicidal state, although she suffered some memory loss and confusion. *Undercurrents* received outstanding reviews from many publications including the *New York Times Book Review* and *The Los Angeles Times*.

Understanding Postpartum Psychosis, by Teresa Twomey, JD with Shoshana Bennett. (Praeger Publishers, 2009) *Understanding Postpartum Psychosis* is one of the few books to date that discusses postpartum bipolar. Teresa Twomey has created an outstanding resource that has been called "the definitive book on postpartum psychosis." Twomey's writing is clear and her research is accurate. Her case studies have been mindfully chosen so that they personalize this often-demonized disorder. Twomey's co-author Dr. Bennett, a top perinatal mental health authority, lends her expertise to the book. Bipolar, peripartum onset (postpartum bipolar disorder) is knowledgeably discussed within *Understanding Postpartum Psychosis*.

BLOGS BY MOMS WITH POST-PARTUM BIPOLAR DISORDER

Birth of a Bipolar Mother / Naissance d'une mère bipolaire
Geneviève Desrochers

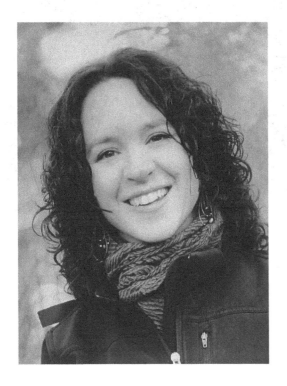

(photo courtesy of Jennifer Campbell)
post-partum-bipolaire.me

Birth of a New Brain—Healing from Postpartum Bipolar Disorder
Dyane Harwood

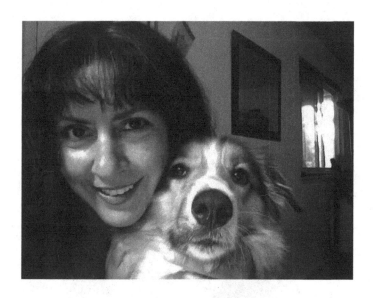

(photo courtesy of Crystal Crafton)
proudlybipolar.wordpress.com

Kitt O'Malley: Love, Live and Learn with Bipolar Disorder
Kitt O'Malley

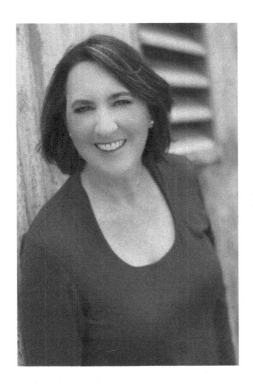

kittomalley.com

Bipolar and Me
Ann Preston Roselle

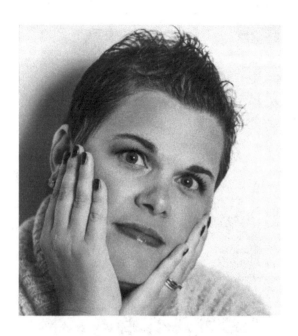

(photo courtesy of Keith Roselle Photography)
bipolarandme.virb.com/about
Learn more about Ann in the remarkable Deconstructing Stigma *campaign at:*
deconstructingstigma.org/stories/?fs=Ann-41

ACKNOWLEDGEMENTS

To the one who started me on the writing path: I'm thankful to my mother Phyllis Leshin for nurturing my love of reading and writing. She gave me *A Wrinkle in Time* by Madeleine L'Engle and *Anne of Green Gables* by L.M. Montgomery, two of the best gifts I've received.

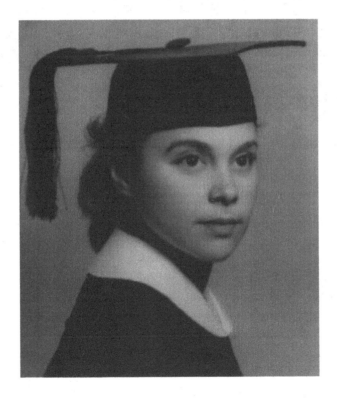

My mother, Phyllis Leshin

To an extraordinary woman who was ahead of her time: My grandmother Frances Nettie Messinger was an incredible role model who made me feel loved and seen.

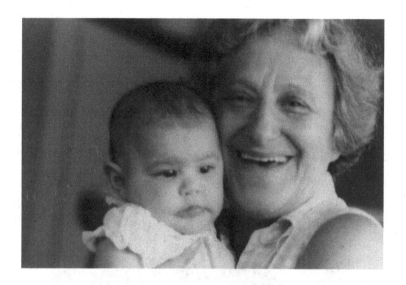

My grandmother, Frances Nettie Messinger

To the publishing team that believed in my book: Thanks to Anthony Ziccardi, Michael Wilson, Billie Brownell, Devon Brown and Beth Dorward of Post Hill Press for giving me the chance to be a Post Hill Press author and for helping the book come to fruition. I'm grateful to designer Vanessa Maynard for creating a cover design that made me and the girls scream. (With delight!)

To the movers, shakers, and story makers: Marie Abanga, Yvette Adams, April Addington, Dr. Mohammad Alsuwaidan, Greg Archer, Dr. Shoshana Bennett, Tim Campen, Chorel Centers, Jim Coffis, Crystal Crafton, Dr. Wendy N. Davis, Dr. Sharon DeVinney, Geneviève Desrochers, Mary Doyle, Christina Dunbar, Teenamarie Flacco, Dr. Raja Gangopadhyay, Maggie and Karma Graham, Lindsay Lipton Gerszt, Syed Afzal Haider, L. E. Henderson, Gabe Howard, Sheryl Isaacs, Dr. Kay Redfield Jamison, Elizabeth Jones, Dr. Shimi Kang, Jenn Larson, Jean Lee, Frances Lefkowitz, Jay Mohr, Kitt O'Malley, Linda Myers, Natachia Barlow Ramsay, Ann Preston Roselle, Joel Sax, Barbara Schweizer, Catherine Segurson, Dr. Verinder Sharma, Bradley Shreve, Allison Strong, Maryann Terhune, Teresa Twomey, Martha Graham-Waldon, Jo Washburn, Salle Webber, and last but not least, Wendy K. Williamson, my writing champion!

To my kindred spirit friends: Suzanne Andersen, Casa Nostra of Ben Lomond, Raffaele Cristallo and Mario Desantis, Aubrey Smith Duerr, Ken, Lisha and Leah Erez and family, Cheantelle Fisher, Mike Freeman, Phil Hebner, Sara Jaesler, Ulla Kelly, Karen Kleiman, Andrea Koenig, Lori Miller, Cori D. Reifman, Brianne Ryan, Carol Stephen, Monika Tessmer, Michelle Ward-Mendoza, and Merry Ruthe Wilson.

To the accomplished mental health experts who believed in me: Dr. Carol Henshaw and Ina.

To the authors whose books helped me escape my turmoil: Madeleine L'Engle, L.M. Montgomery, Anthony Bourdain, and SARK.

To the artists and musicians whose creativity fed my soul and gave me hope: Adam Ant, Toni Childs, Chris Difford, Dave Dobbyn, Thomas Dolby, Neil and Tim Finn, Paul Hester, Howard Jones, Paul Baker Jones, Annie Lennox, Aimee Mann, Roland Orzabal, Nick Seymour, Curt Smith, and Glenn Tilbrook,

To my best friend who sat on my foot during the writing of this book: My Scotch collie Lucy.

To my father: Dad, how I wish you were here to celebrate with me. I hope you're seeing this excitement from some fantastic place.

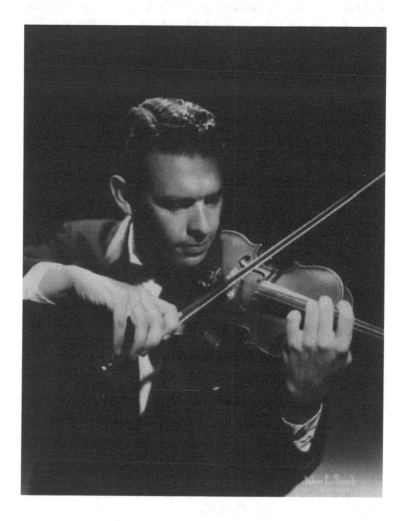

My father, Richard David Leshin

ABOUT THE AUTHOR

Dyane Harwood holds a B.A. in English and American Literature from the University of California at Santa Cruz. A freelance writer for two decades, she has interviewed the bestselling authors Dr. Kay Redfield Jamison, Anthony Bourdain, and SARK. In 2007, Harwood was diagnosed with postpartum bipolar disorder (bipolar disorder, peripartum onset.) Her memoir *Birth of a New Brain, Healing from Postpartum Bipolar Disorder* is the first book to discuss a woman's experience with this rare form of bipolar disorder and overlooked postpartum mood disorder. Harwood has been profiled in *The Huffington Post* about her postpartum mental health advocacy. PsychCentral honored Harwood as a Mental Health Hero, and the International Bipolar Foundation featured her as a "Story of Hope and Recovery." Harwood has written about postpartum bipolar disorder for *The Huffington Post*, *The Mighty*, *Anchor Magazine*, Postpartum Support International, Postpartum Progress, the International Society for Bipolar Disorders and the Stigma Fighters Anthology. She founded a chapter of the Depression and Bipolar Support Alliance (DBSA) and facilitated free support groups for mothers with mood disorders for nine years. Dyane lives in Ben Lomond, California, with her two daughters, husband, and Scotch collie.